an Happiness

JAMES E. HUSTON, M.D., F.A.C.O.G.

☑® Facts On File, Inc.

MENOPAUSE: A GUIDE TO HEALTH AND HAPPINESS

Facts On File, Inc.
11 Penn Plaza
New York NY 10001

Library of Congress Cataloging-in-Publication Data
Huston, James E.
Menopause : a guide to health and happiness / by James E. Huston.
p. cm.
Includes bibliographical references and index.
ISBN 0-8160-3675-6 (hardcover).—ISBN 0-8160-3693-4 (pbk.)
1. Menopause—Popular works. I. Title.
RG186.H786 1998
618.1'75—dc21 97-36897

Facts On File books are available at special discounts when purchased in bulk quantities for businesses, associations, institutions or sales promotions. Please call our Special Sales Department in New York at (212) 967-8800 or (800) 322-8755.

You can find Facts On File on the World Wide Web at http://www.factsonfile.com

Text design by Cathy Rincon
Cover design by Semadar Megged
Layout by Robert Yaffe
Illustrations by Jeremy Eagle

Printed in the United States of America

MP FOF 10 9 8 7 6 5 4 3 2 1

This book is printed on acid-free paper.

To Toria. Who else?

We lived it together.

CONTENTS 🍃

ACKNOWLEDGMENTS

My special thanks to those women (and men) who read my manuscript and offered their criticisms and comments. I was flattered by your interest, encouraged by your positive comments, and enlightened by your criticism. You have done me an invaluable service. In addition, my profound gratitude goes to the thousands of patients who entrusted me to teach them and who, in turn, taught me.

AUTHOR'S NOTE

To write about menopause as a physician, and a male physician at that, seemed initially quite daunting. Most authors currently writing on the subject are professional writers and/or women. Nonetheless, I decided to jump into the fray. My decision stems from several different observations and experiences.

After three decades of medical practice, and consultations with many thousands of women who were menopausal or about to be menopausal, I found that the level of knowledge about this natural occurrence is quite low, and not increasing. Old myths (femininity is over, for example) persist and they are multiplying—all this in the "Information Age." Those of us in the information dissemination business had been doing a pretty poor job, it seemed to me. My personal efforts to educate the women who trusted me to guide them generally succeeded in arming them with sufficient information to make educated choices about menopause, but these mini-courses were all one-on-one. Individual instruction is fine, of course, but the number of women who require this information is increasing constantly. With the advent of the women of the 76 million "boomer generation" reaching the age of menopause, that number is sure to swell. As a gynecologist, I had been swimming against the tide.

The references available to the 46 million women over age 45 who need information about menopause typically are books, health care educators, print and broadcast media, lectures, videos, schools, seminars, mothers, friends, focus groups and the like. That is an impressive array of resources but, in spite of this, ignorance about menopause seems little diminished. We have done a terrible job of informing the public and of making menopause an acceptable part of midlife, as well as an acceptable topic of discussion. Thus, this natural and inevitable change remains largely a closed subject. It does not make the evening TV news or the newspapers; our youth-oriented film industry shuns it; and you don't hear it discussed at dinner parties. Physicians and other health care givers are frequently too busy, or not themselves well enough informed, to provide necessary information. The dozens of books currently in print are often well conceived but sometimes reveal flaws such as the author's bias about what constitutes valid management of menopausal problems, complaints against the medical establishment for not knowing more than it does, tons of nonessential information, writing so scholarly and dry that the reader is put off, and misinterpretations of medical data and erroneous conclusions. All this literature is in some way useful, flaws and all, because it puts menopause out there for discussion, though not nearly to the extent needed. So, I reasoned, maybe I *should* write a book.

I regard menopause not as the beginning of impending decline but as an opportunity for a woman to review her health status and start on a beneficial health program. It is a signal for the future and a chance to become educated on how to manage aging successfully. From the onset of menopause, at least one-third of life remains to be lived and these years can be joyous and productive if knowledge of this normal life event leads to a healthful living pattern. Women need to know this.

Events in my personal life also impelled me to write this book. I had a minor stroke in the summer of 1994. I recovered from it in a few weeks, but it convinced me to stop active medical practice, since a sudden recurrence might jeopardize a mother or her baby in my care. Since then, I have been "smelling the roses," paying a great deal more attention to the joy of being alive. With my wife Victoria's unstinting support, her improving our diet and reorganizing our exercise routines, we have evolved a new and healthier lifestyle. "Toria" herself has recently become menopausal and has gone through many of the events and problems discussed in this book. I have experienced them with her. So, with my background in women's health care and my wife's firsthand experience of menopause, in addition to our coping with the above situations together, I felt that I was well qualified to write on this subject.

Considering all of the above, I concluded that the greatest number of women could be best served if a compact guide was written. It would need to be honest, up-to-date, comprehensive without being tedious, and easy to understand. Most important, it would have to consider the whole woman and her milieu—not just her anatomy, her physiology, her psyche.

What follows is the result. My fondest hope is that the natural midlife transition we call menopause can become a widely understood and accepted part of life and that this book will further that goal. Millions of women (and men) need and desire to know the who, what, where, when, how, and why of this relatively untalked-about and poorly understood life event.

SECTION I

PERIMENOPAUSE

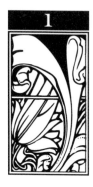

BACKGROUND TALK

A Flaw in the Grand Plan? . . . Women Are Living Longer

For the first thousands of years that humans walked the earth, women did not live much beyond menopause. Other primates (monkeys, apes) are the same, reproducing right up to the end of life. That seems to have been nature's grand plan. *But* in the last century or so, of our thousands of centuries on this planet, we started living longer. We ate better, clothed ourselves better, and housed ourselves better. We had better medicines and vaccines, better sewage disposal, better working conditions, and many other new things that together contributed to our longer life span. Women have benefited somewhat more than men: Women live a few years longer. Life expectancy for American women is 81 years; however a woman who is 65 can expect another 18½ years.

Living longer was not part of the original plan perhaps; but that is, nonetheless, how it is going. Something that did *not* change however, is the age of menopause. For the most part, the reproductive phase of a woman's life has always ended in her 40s. In some cultures it is a few years earlier. In the United States it is about age 51 or 52—somewhat older than at the beginning of the current century. To the everlasting joy of their partners, women are no longer dying off as soon as menopause has occurred. As a matter of fact, women live fully one-third of their lives *after* their reproductive era has ended. With such a divergence from nature's plan in only a century or so, there has not been nearly enough experience, or science, to guide women in how best to live these extra years. Would you call that a flaw? Should the "Grand Planner" reconvene the committee?

It could get even trickier too. Geneticists and other scientists are busy mapping the human genome. They are locating each gene and defining what it does for us, or *to* us. The gene, or genes, that control aging will eventually be understood, as will the genes that cause cancer, heart disease, and many other fatal illnesses. Genetic engineering will favorably alter the course of many of these conditions. More people will be alive as a result. In addition, we could all live longer if the geneticists are correct in their estimate that humans can probably live 120 to 140 years. That translates to perhaps 70 to 90 years of a woman's life yet to live *after* menopause. At present, however, women will live an average of 30 years beyond menopause; so let us deal with nature's little oversight as it now exists.

Definitions . . . Just a Few

Menopause means the natural and permanent cessation of menstrual periods. The word comes from the Greek *men* (month) + *pausis* (cessation, pause). Menopause, then, is actually a point in time rather than the entire era after cessation of periods, as we commonly refer to it. I doubt if the truly accurate use of the term will be adopted by most people, since it is so well established as referring to the entire postreproductive time of life. Menopause is not a disease, so it does not require a cure. It is the natural aging of the reproductive system. Our interest and concern with menopause is that it speeds up the aging of other parts of your body such as the heart, bones, muscle, skin, genital anatomy, and brain.

Perimenopause, if strictly defined, refers to the few years preceding and just after menopause; but we more commonly apply the term differently. It has come to mean those years between normal menstrual functioning and cessation of menstrual periods. It would be more accurate to call this era the *transitional period.* This transition can be many years in length, and actually starts as early as the mid- to late 30s; but generally it encompasses the mid-40s to early 50s age range when menstrual periods and cycles become irregular.

Postmenopause refers to the entire length of time after menstrual periods have permanently stopped.

Climacteric is a less commonly used term referring to the collection of events and symptoms that occur between the mid-40s and mid-50s. It encompasses perimenopause, menopause, and the first few years of post-menopause.

Other terms will be defined later in the book, and the glossary in the back will help you with any unfamiliar words you encounter.

The Numbers Are Amazing

There are now over 46 million women in the United States over the age of 45. By the turn of the century, one-third of our country's women will be over 50. More than 16 million women are age 45 to 55, the age bracket in which menopausal information is the most critically needed. But guess what's next: the baby boomer generation of 76 million souls born between 1946 and 1964, about half of whom are women of course, *and* the oldest of whom are already menopausal. According to the National Council on Aging, the first boomer turned 50 on January 1, 1996, and that will continue unabated at the rate of 1 woman every 15 seconds for a full 10 years.

Unlike the generations that preceded them, the boomers have been a more open, more inquisitive, and more "take charge" group. They are information omnivores. A good example of an outcome of their energy and drive is the way they changed child birthing in the United States: natural birthing, fathers in attendance, a family event.

The predecessors of the boomers were more or less silent about menopause. They were fearful of it, shamed by it, and plagued by inadequate information as well as by misinformation. The coming millions can be expected to grab it, shake it, read about it, talk about it, and finally get menopause out of the closet so that *all* concerned can benefit from the available information. In my view, that's terrific, and I hope this book will be useful to them.

OK, So What Happens?

The basic event in the perimenopausal transition to menopause is that you start running out of eggs. This results in your ovaries being unable to produce adequate amounts of *estrogen* and *progesterone*, the major female sex hormones. Specifics are in the next chapter. When ovarian function slows, a cascade of succeeding symptoms and events is set in motion: irregular periods, hot flashes, sleep disruption, diminished sexual desire, short-term memory loss, mood swings, cessation of periods, bone loss (osteoporosis), heart disease, vascular (blood vessel) disease, diminished vaginal secretions, skin dryness and wrinkling, breast shrinking and sagging, frequent urinary tract infections, and other problems too; but this covers most of it. Well let's hope so.

As you can see, these hormone deficiencies affect your heart, blood vessels, bones, brain, genital organs, and skin. All of these changes don't happen at once, thank heavens, nor does each and every one of them happen to every woman. They happen in a gradual and unpredictable fashion, turning up as surprises along the way.

As troublesome as the physical symptoms are, the psychological, social, and sexual changes can be even more daunting. Consider where a woman is in life when nature pulls the rug from beneath her. Mothers have completed their child rearing, career women are at the apex of their power, professionals like teachers, lawyers, and physicians are at their most effective career stage, writers and artists have matured, workers of every stripe are ready for smoother times ahead. Then, for no apparent reason, a healthy and vigorous woman starts feeling like a wet paper towel . . . limp, no energy. Hot flashes intrude on daily routines and cause sleep disruption. You get cranky about stuff that never bothered you before. Sex is less desirable. Moods gyrate all over the map. Clothes fit a little too snug. Waves of unexplainable sadness wash over you. "I can't remember what I did with the blasted car keys!" Sound familiar?

About this time an aging parent may become dependent. Your partner may develop a health problem or have a crisis of his own, such as retirement or loss of his job. One of the kids (most likely a son) wants to move back home. Surveys have shown that the "return to the nest syndrome" is much more frustrating than the "empty nest syndrome." You become a grandmother, and your unmarried daughter plus child want to move in.

What's going on here? Without much prior notice, this magnificent human being, who has so masterfully nurtured and orchestrated her family, her marriage, her occupation, and her world, has lost control. It is perplexing at first because nothing really unmanageable (by her previous standards) has happened. Panic starts when she cannot regain control; this is quickly followed by outrage at the injustice of nature's heartless blow.

"Am I to be old and useless now?" "I don't look young anymore, so who will love me?" "My credibility is gone." "Who needs me anymore?" "From where will my strokes come?" A thousand more doubts surface, all of which make you wonder if you will ultimately become invisible. What an utter, total, absolute, and unmitigated CALAMITY! Well, don't flip out over this. There's good news.

OK, So What Can I Do about It?

The one thing you can *not* do about menopause is prevent it. It is a natural part of the aging process, and a transition through which all women (no exceptions) will pass in their middle years. Many, if not most, women will initially deny that the symptoms they are having are related to the "change of life." Gail Sheehy, in her groundbreaking book *The Silent Passage*, found in her interviews that women are afraid to know that menopause could be affecting them; but on the other hand, they secretly and desperately want to know all about it.

An extensive menu of management choices is available to relieve the symptoms and avert the hazards posed by this midlife hormonal change. Included are hormone replacement therapy (HRT), alternative medical therapies, stress management techniques, and improved fitness involving nutrition and exercise. Section III of this book is devoted to the details of these therapies and lifestyle changes.

As mentioned earlier, most women do not develop all of the symptoms and problems listed. There is a nearly unlimited variation from one woman to the next, and that makes it obvious that each woman who seeks help must be dealt with as an individual. No cookbook treatment plan works. Some make the transition with hardly a ripple of difficulty, while some are devastated. The majority are able, with personal endeavor and third-party help, to overcome the transitory problems. *Transitory* is an important word here because most of the disagreeable symptoms (hot flashes, irritability, short-term memory loss, fatigue) are indeed temporary. There are therapies and lifestyle techniques that can control these disagreeable symptoms; but it is also known that they will go away in time, even if you do nothing.

Some of the problems will not go away no matter how long you wait. Menopause is not a disease process, but the changes in your body which can result from the absence of your female hormones can be very threatening to your health. The most serious of these is the risk of heart attack and stroke. Bone loss, called *osteoporosis*, can result in fractures that may be a life threat also. Certain cancer risks (breast, uterus, colon) are changed after menopause. These are not transitory or temporary problems. Many of the increased risks can be easily averted or at least favorably modified by active, positive management.

Management choice is a major theme of this book. What is right for one woman may not be for another; this is why it is important for you to become informed regarding what is available. Whether a management regimen is effective and safe must also be considered. While no management plan is risk free, the greatest risk to your health after menopause is to do nothing. There are no racial, cultural, or geographic barriers to menopause. It is universal. This brief guide is about getting through and emerging from this transition intact, healthy, and prepared for your great life ahead.

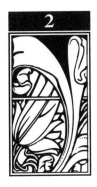

PERIMENOPAUSE: HOW IT HAPPENS

Now for some physiology and a little anatomy. Wait, wait, wait . . . don't close the book. I'll use plain language and diagrams. It won't take long, and there won't be any quiz at the end. I want you to know how the female hormonal cycle works, so you can understand what goes on when it doesn't work. Then I'll show how you can tell whether you are, or are not, perimenopausal.

The Lifetime Hormone Curve

Menarche is the term for the onset of the first menstrual period, and *menopause* is for the last one. Both of these events is a point in time. It is important to understand that the events leading up to the beginning of the reproductive era, the reproductive era itself, and the postreproductive era are a spectrum. It is a time curve of ascending hormone production, then a plateau of hormone production, and finally a decline of hormone production. Figure 2-1 illustrates this. The first part of the curve results in the development of female sex characteristics like pubic hair, breasts, and menstrual periods. The last part sees a decline of these characteristics and constitutes perimenopause, menopause, and postmenopause.

Perimenopause has typically been regarded as those few years between the middle 40s and the early 50s when symptoms and signs of estrogen decline become apparent. As can be seen in Figure 2-1, however, a woman's lifetime peak of estrogen production is in her late 20s. A slow decline in total monthly estrogen output begins at that time. The levels are quite adequate for maintaining her reproductive capability and sexual responsiveness for many years.

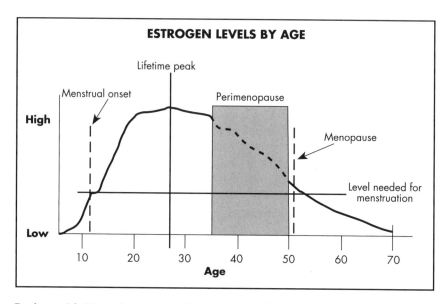

ESTROGEN LEVELS BY AGE

By her mid-30s, subtle signs of estrogen decline, such as minor changes in menstrual periods, may begin. It is unlikely that these changes would be noticed. After age 40, the signs and symptoms of estrogen deficiency become more noticeable. These will be discussed in the next chapter. The point here is that perimenopause covers a 10–15 year span, rather than those 4–6 years after her mid-40s.

Now Some Basics . . . The Cycle Is Just a Daisy Chain

The basic information about perimenopause and menopause will be much easier to understand if you first know how the menstrual cycle works normally. The cycle is a feedback mechanism. It involves three hormone-producing glands working in concert: the *hypothalamus* in your brain, the *pituitary* also in your brain, and your *ovaries*. Each of these three glands produces a variety of hormones (chemical messengers) which enter your bloodstream and are then taken to their various target organs. We will only consider the hormones associated with the menstrual cycle.

The hypothalamus, pituitary, and ovaries form a sort of daisy chain and communicate with each other through their hormone messengers. As a starting point, we will enter the cycle at day one, the first day of a menstrual period. At this point of the cycle, female hormone levels of estrogen and progesterone are low. At day one of the cycle your hypothalamus becomes aware of the low hormone levels and starts sending a releasing hormone to your pituitary called *gonadotropin releasing hormone* (GnRH). This hormone tells your pituitary to release its two hormones targeted for your ovaries called *follicle stimulating hormone* (FSH) and *luteinizing hormone* (LH). Their message to your ovaries is that they should mature some egg follicles and start producing more female hormones (estrogen and progesterone). Ovulation will be coming up soon, and an egg needs to be ready in case any sperm might be in the neighborhood to start a pregnancy.

A few more items are in order before we finish describing the cycle. Estrogen is produced by the ovarian cells in the follicle wall. Progesterone is produced there too, but most of it is produced after the egg in the follicle is released. Estrogen and progesterone together are responsible for thickening the lining of your uterus to prepare it for a pregnancy if the egg becomes fertilized. After ovulation, the follicle is turned into a structure called the *corpus luteum* which makes progesterone plus another glycoprotein chemical called *inhibin*. There is some disagreement about inhibin's function, but it is thought that inhibin plays a role in regulating FSH production in the pituitary (i.e., it inhibits FSH) and thus plays an important role in cycling. Back to the cycle . . .

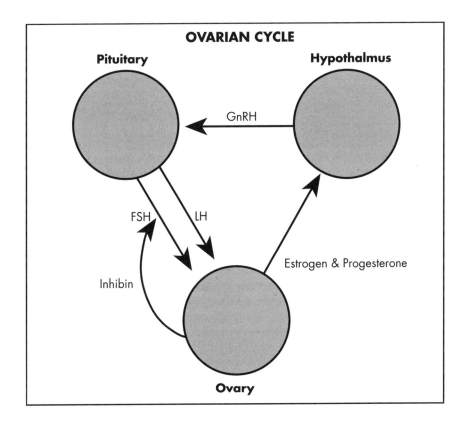

OVARIAN CYCLE

Pituitary

Hypothalmus

GnRH

FSH LH

Inhibin

Estrogen & Progesterone

Ovary

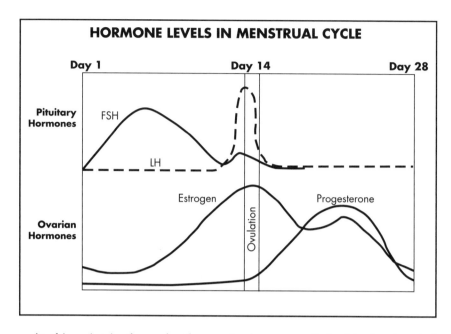

HORMONE LEVELS IN MENSTRUAL CYCLE

Day 1   Day 14   Day 28

Pituitary Hormones

FSH

LH

Estrogen

Ovulation

Progesterone

Ovarian Hormones

At this point in the cycle, the ovaries have complied with the chemical messages from the pituitary. Ovulation has taken place; the ovarian hormones, plus inhibin, are out there in the bloodstream. That message gets back to the hypothalamus and to the pituitary, both of which are satisfied that the cycling system is working perfectly. So, the hypothalamus takes the heat off the pituitary by reducing GnRH, and the pituitary takes the heat off the ovaries by reducing FSH and LH. The ovaries respond by dropping their output of estrogen, progesterone, and inhibin. Figure 2-2 shows the interplay of all these hormonal messages. The net result of all these messages and responses is that the lining of your uterus, called the *endometrium*, is no longer supported by the female hormones, and it is shed—a menstrual period happens.

Now the hypothalamus and pituitary become aware that the ovaries are down there in the pelvis taking a breather, because the bloodstream is showing low levels of estrogen, progesterone, and inhibin. So they say, "Good job group; but let's take it again from the top," and the cycle starts over. All this takes about four weeks. In Figure 2-3, you can see how the levels of the pituitary and ovarian hormones rise and fall during this 28-day cycle.

The Perimenopausal Process (Ovaries from Fetus to Forties)

During fetal life, ovaries contain up to 7 million egg follicles. By birth, the count is down to about 2 million. This amazing reduction in follicles occurs over a period of about 20 weeks during pregnancy, as the growing ovary pushes the surface follicles out into the abdominal cavity of the fetus (Speroff 1989). By puberty, there are only about 400,000 left; but that is still plenty, because you will ovulate only about 400 times during your reproductive years. At ovulation, as many as 1,000 follicles are ready to release their ova, but usually only one makes the grade. The rest then shrink away. Multiple pregnancies can happen when multiple ovulations occur (fraternal twins) or when a single fertilized egg splits in two (identical twins). Humans are not well designed for litters, however, and single egg release is the usual result. By age 40, only a few thousand follicles remain to produce estrogen and progesterone. As the follicles continue to decrease in number, so does the production of inhibin. Eventually, not enough hormone is produced to prepare the endometrium of the uterus anymore. As a result, no shedding occurs, and periods stop. This gradual slowdown is the perimenopausal transition. The changes that perimenopause causes in your body and in your life are covered later. For now, my purpose is to explain how it comes about.

Variations on the Theme . . . If the Daisy Chain Gets Broken

As elegant and well designed as the menstrual cycle is, it is not without flaws. A number of situations can disrupt it. If any of the three glands (hypothalamus, pituitary, ovary) of the daisy chain gets sick or knocked out for some reason, the chain is broken and cycling stops. The most visible end point of the broken chain is no menstrual periods. If that happens, the question to ask and get answered is, Which of the three is the culprit? There is a whole battery of tests that can reliably find the culprit, but some simple observations can usually point in the right direction, while saving time and expense.

+ The hypothalamus is commonly suppressed by outside situations such as severe chronic stress, starvation (anorexia, bulimia), excessive exercise (common in Olympic athletes), and birth control pills.
+ The pituitary is a bit more subtle because its problems can come from an old head injury, a slow growing tumor in the pituitary, severe blood loss with cardiovascular shock, and other hormone disturbances. Often the finger gets pointed at the pituitary only when it is known that the other two on the daisy chain are OK. Then specific pituitary tests are run.

✦ When rounding up the usual suspects, the ovaries are, of course, included. Topping the list of questions regarding no menstrual periods is always, Did an ovum and a sperm get it together? If the pregnancy test is negative, though, look to other things. If you are 50 years old, your periods are irregular or absent, you are having hot flashes, are moody and irritable, can't sleep, and can't remember what you did with the blasted car keys, then perimenopause or menopause deserves serious consideration. Less common problems such as ovarian tumors should also be considered, but pregnancy and menopause are the most frequent sources of absent menstrual periods.

OK, So Prove It . . . Diagnosis

Diagnosing perimenopause and menopause is a process. The process is initiated by consulting a health care professional who is qualified to help you. This can be a gynecologist, an internist, a family practitioner, or a women's health clinic. The initial obligation of your consultant is to *think* that your situation could be arising from your being perimenopausal. Arriving at this first step happens only after listening to you, evaluating your current life, and knowing about your past health. Skillful professionals also pay attention to your nonverbal communication such as facial expression, vocal tones, and body language. Physicians refer to this process as "taking a medical history." Physical examination is also an important adjunct in arriving at the right answer to your problem; but hearing about it and *listening* to what one is hearing are crucial. A few examples of the importance of listening follow:

✦ If you have been missing periods, are having hot flashes, are tense and grumpy, can't remember where you put the blasted car keys, and are 48 years old, then your ovaries (and perimenopause) are definitely suspect.

✦ If you have been missing periods, are tense and grumpy, can't remember where you put the blasted car keys, but are a 19-year-old college freshman on birth control pills, and away from home for the first time, then a stressed hypothalamus is a more logical consideration.

✦ If you have been missing periods, are tense and grumpy, can't remember where you put the blasted car keys, and are a world-class athlete who runs 85 miles per week, again the hypothalamus makes more sense to investigate than your ovaries.

So far, you have not been examined or had a lab test. If you have been listened to, however, and your complete story *heard*, you are already going in the right direction for a correct diagnosis. Once it has become suspicious that your ovaries have diminished their normal function, it still remains to be shown that this is indeed the case. In the past, this was done by testing your blood level of FSH. The rationale for doing an FSH test was based on the fact that when your ovaries are not producing enough estrogen, your pituitary puts out more FSH in an attempt to get your flagging ovaries to respond. And if your ovaries do not respond, the pituitary thinks, "Maybe they didn't get my message," and it sends out more FSH, and more, and more, and more. Pretty soon there is an abnormally high level of FSH in your bloodstream. During the childbearing years, a normal FSH level is under 10 mIU/ml (milli International Units per milliliter). When it gets over 20–30 mIU/ml, the suspicion of ovarian slowdown is confirmed, and the closer it gets to 40, the closer you are to menopause.

Having said all that about diagnosing perimenopause with FSH testing, I must now tell you that it is no longer being used for this purpose. The reasons are twofold. First, it is an expensive test. Second, during perimenopause your ovarian production of hormones is subject to ups and downs. If your FSH level is tested during an "up" month, it will be normal even though you may be truly perimenopausal. It takes two consecutive months of abnormal FSH results to make the diagnosis, so you may end up doing multiple tests before a confident diagnosis can be established. Reliance on elevated FSH levels can therefore be an expensive method of chasing a diagnosis of perimenopause.

Direct testing of your estrogen blood level is not used to establish a diagnosis of perimenopause either. The normal level has traditionally been thought to vary from about 90 pg/ml (picograms per milliliter) at the beginning of a cycle, to around 500 at midcycle. In the past, an estradiol (estrogen) level of less than 60 was regarded as evidence of estrogen deficiency. It has now been shown that as many an one-third of women with normal cycles will have an estradiol level as low as 20 at the beginning of each cycle. This observation makes relying on a level below 60 useless for establishing a diagnosis of estrogen deficiency.

For these reasons, laboratory testing to prove perimenopause is no longer being used. Instead, most physicians give a trial of hormone replacement if you are having typical symptoms and signs of estrogen decline. This can be in the form of estrogen and progesterone supplements, or low dose birth control pills for women who are still in the reproductive era of life. This is discussed more extensively in Chapter 12 on hormone replacement. If you fail to respond positively, other causes of your symptoms, such as hypothyroidism, must be investigated.

Summing Up

Perimenopause represents the time frame between your middle 30s to your early 50s when production of your female sex hormones is declining. It signals the normal aging of your reproductive system. This chapter has shown you how and why it occurs. The next chapter will show you what you can expect from perimenopause, in your life and in your body.

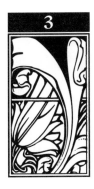

PERIMENOPAUSE: AS IT HAPPENS

The signs and symptoms of perimenopause are discussed in this chapter. These are the high profile changes that can get to you and alter your life quite noticeably. The lower profile, and more health threatening, changes are mentioned but will be covered in depth in later chapters. You will find a menu of available management options and a discussion of the helping role that men can play. Yes it's true, men can help.

Now, Perimenopause More Specifically

SYMPTOMS HAPPEN

The signs and symptoms of perimenopause that most commonly occur are menstrual irregularities, hot flashes, unexplained fatigue, sleep disruption, mood alterations, and short-term memory loss. These are the high profile, early changes, which are easily recognized. The low profile, later changes include beginning of increased risk for heart attacks and stroke, escalation of bone loss (osteoporosis), unintended pregnancy (which does not stay low profile for long, of course), changing cancer risks, thinning and dryness of the vaginal lining (can be an early change), thinning of the skin, urethra and bladder, and diminished sexual desire (also can be an early change). Let us first consider the high profile signs and symptoms.

Menstrual Irregularity

During perimenopause, your menstrual periods can vary all over the map: too much, too little, too often, not often enough, and none. The typical pattern for menstrual change in the perimenopausal transition is a normal menstrual period, in a cycle that is shorter than the usual 28 days. This is followed by a period of time when your ovaries are not releasing eggs, and the cycle lengthens to more than 28 days, sometimes with more prolonged menstrual bleeding. Eventually periods are skipped from time to time and, ultimately, they stop. This is the average pattern but it can vary dramatically.

The medical term for "too much," or heavy bleeding, is *hypermenorrhea*; gushing is what we are talking about here. It happens because you have not been ovulating regularly and your ovaries did not produce a normal amount of progesterone. This hormone is responsible for changing the lining of your uterus so it can be easily impregnated, or easily shed. If you are getting estrogen only, the lining becomes a bit thicker and it sheds less readily, resulting in heavier bleeding.

Another early sign is "not often enough." The fancy medical term for this is *oligomenorrhea*, but the more common phraseology is "Oh my gosh, I've missed my period!" . . . and many other unprintable exclamatory variations. Even though your ability to get pregnant has been declining slowly since your 30s, a pregnancy test still tops the list of things to do *now*.

"Too little," or scanty bleeding, is called *hypomenorrhea*. Not many perimenopausal women are outraged by this turn of events. It simply represents reduced hormone effectiveness and a thinner endometrium that requires less shedding.

"Too often" is a bit more of a hassle, I'm certain you will agree. This initially happens because of a shortening of the first half of the cycle. Later, when ovulation is no longer happening, progesterone is no longer produced in normal amounts and a "no-pattern" type of uterine bleeding may ensue. It is called *polymenorrhea*, or more commonly *dysfunctional uterine bleeding*. The prolonged absence of ovulation causes a buildup of the thickness of the endometrium by estrogen, which is unopposed by progesterone. Not knowing when your period is coming is guaranteed to make you bonkers.

Amenorrhea, better known as "none at all," gradually develops after several years, and then this perimenopausal menstrual irregularity episode is over. Only 10% of women have an abrupt cessation of menstrual periods—not fair perhaps, but that is what you can expect.

Finally, please do not ignore these menstrual changes. Get a consultation, because sometimes they can be the result of a more serious problem than perimenopausal change. In addition, it is usually possible to control the more aggravating forms of irregular bleeding with hormone supplementation or low dose birth control pills (covered later in this section).

Table 3-1		
HOT FLASHES IN AMERICAN WOMEN		
Duration	**Percent**	
1–2 years	Up to 75%	
5 years	20–50%	
Indefinitely	10%	

Hot Flashes, Hot Flushes, and Vasomotor Instability

All three of these terms refer to the same process, but each describe a slightly different aspect of the experience. The most commonly used is *hot flash*, so let's stick with that. The hot flash is one of the hallmarks or defining symptoms of perimenopause and postmenopause. Dr. Fredi Kronenberg's 1990 study reported about 85% of American women experience hot flashes in widely varying intensities and duration. Table 3-1 summarizes this for you.

The Massachusetts Women's Health Study revealed that hot flashes occurred in about 10% of women during the perimenopausal transition, rose to 50% after cessation of menstrual periods, and dropped back to 20% within four years after menopause.

THE HOT FLASH REVEALED

A typical hot flash has a preceding aura lasting about a minute. During the aura you may notice anxiety or dread, as well as increased heart rate, dizziness, or weakness. This is immediately followed by flushing of the upper body, head, and neck accompanied by sweating of these areas. The skin becomes reddened and skin temperature rises by as much as seven degrees as a result of the increased blood flow. The feeling of body heat during the flush is often described as quite intense. Some women say it feels like their makeup is raised about an inch off their face. One woman said: "These are not hot flashes, they're power surges." Chilling often results from the perspiring skin as evaporation begins, a normal consequence of the body's heat release mechanisms. The flushing phase of a hot flash usually lasts about five minutes but can rarely go as long as an hour.

HOW BAD ARE THEY?

Hot flashes vary from one woman to the next. One woman may describe them as mild and easily borne sensations, while the next may be devastated by their frequency and intensity. Kronenberg reported in 1993 that only 10%–15% of women find hot flashes debilitating. Frequency ranges from every 10–15 minutes (not common, but a real cross to bear when it happens) to rare occurrences. One to four a day, and/or night is more common. Most of the time, the feeling of heat is inappropriate to what is going on around you, for example, you are the only one at the dinner party who is sweating profusely.

One of the most disturbing aspects of hot flashes is that they occur more commonly at night than during the day. Sleep disruption occurs during the aura, and you awaken to be greeted by the flush and profuse sweating. This is soon followed by discarded blankets and roused partners. Complete recovery may take as long as half an hour, but now you, or both of you, are wide awake. Most observers agree that disturbed sleep is the primary cause of other common perimenopausal symptoms such as fatigue, moodiness, irritability, short-term memory loss, and impaired concentration.

WHAT CAUSES THIS OUTRAGE?

The exact cause of hot flashes is not completely understood. They apparently occur because of disturbed coordination between the hypothalamus (your body's thermostat) and the *autonomic nervous system* which controls heat conservation and heat release. Diminished estrogen effect seems to be a major underlying cause of this failure of coordination. The net result is that the hypothalamus changes its "set point." This signals the autonomic nervous system to change the heat release mechanism. Then blood vessels (under the command and control of the autonomic nervous system) get temporarily out of whack. The blood vessels dilate, bringing large quantities of blood to your skin for cooling, and your body's heat release mechanisms inappropriately go ape. Hot flashes may occur more commonly at night because during sleep the hypothalamus is less occupied with other regulatory activities. With less estrogen in your system, it just decides to start toying with the thermostat. Women on hormone replacement therapy found that taking their estrogen at bedtime eliminates or drastically reduces night flushing.

Epinephrine (adrenaline) levels are increased during a hot flash. This accounts for the anxious feeling during the aura, as well as the increased heart rate and stepped-up blood flow. Although estrogen reliably relieves hot flashes in over 90% of women, no studies have been completed on a method of controlling epinephrine release. Something like that could be a possible alternative for controlling hot flashes in women who cannot take estrogen.

In perimenopausal women who are still having menstrual periods as well as hot flashes, fluctuating levels of estrogen are thought to be the source. A more recent additional theory is that a poorer quality of estrogen is being produced by the ovary's aging follicles. This means the estrogen is less usable.

Other health conditions in menstruating women can mimic hot flashes. These include diabetes, hyperthyroidism, pheochromocytoma (an adrenal tumor), carcinoid (a tumor in the appendix), leukemia, pancreatic tumors, and alcoholism. So you cannot assume your ovaries are at fault whenever hot flashes occur. The hot flash is also a common psychosomatic symptom. In these situations, it is reasonable to have FSH testing to prove estrogen deficiency before embarking upon a replacement regimen or other options.

GETTING A HANDLE ON THEM

Hormone replacement therapy (HRT) most reliably controls hot flashes in two to six weeks. HRT, aerobic exercise, and alternative therapies are all helpful, and they are fully discussed in Section III.

Prevention of hot flashes, or at least decreasing the chances of a hot flash, may be possible by avoiding hot weather, hot food, hot drinks, hot clothes, hot beds, hot rooms, hot tubs, alcohol, and stress. All of these situations trigger hot flashes. Eating a large meal can also trigger one because digestion brings large amounts of blood into your abdomen. This raises your core temperature and unleashes your heat releasing mechanisms. Acute or chronic stress from any cause is very commonly associated with hot flashes, so it deserves serious attempts to control it.

Nutritional status plays a role in hot flashes, since it is known that women who are vegetarians or underweight have more severe menopausal symptoms. This is related to the fact that fatty tissue can be converted to a weak estrogen, called *estrone*, by a process called *aromatization*. This is not an endorsement for obesity, but a few extra calories might be helpful if your body habitus is fashion-modelesque.

Exercise is a *very* good hot flash modulator. If possible, go for a walk when you get one. Regular exercise is much more efficient than the occasional walk, though. In a 1982 study of scheduled aerobic exercise, more than half of perimenopausal and postmenopausal women reported diminished hot flashes, *and* their estrogen levels increased (Wallace 1982). Besides, going out for a walk at 3:30 A.M. does not have a lot of appeal for most; and it may really bomb if you ask your partner to accompany you. Nutrition and exercise are covered in Chapter 14.

Cognitive Changes . . . Brain Drain

"I'm falling apart." "They may take me away." "He dropped that third peanut shell and I went absolutely ballistic." "And I can't remember where I put the blasted car keys." "Moody? *Me* moody? Now just what the hell do you mean by that?" (Spoken while standing with feet spread and hands on hips).

In her book *The Silent Passage*, Gail Sheehy comments: "At forty you can't read the numbers in the phone book. At fifty you can't remember them." This is a telling remark on a common complaint in perimenopause . . . short-term memory loss. It is just one of a constellation of symptoms involving brain function. Thinking gets slower. Logic gets fuzzy. Vocabulary selection becomes labored. You start to interject a pithy thought into a stimulating conversation and forget your point halfway through. Frustration is an understatement. An in-control and smooth functioning woman at the peak of her powers and upon whom many have come to depend (children, partner, coworkers, parents) has seemingly come apart like a cheap watch.

There is no question that the brain and its cognitive functions are affected by female hormone withdrawal. Moodiness, irritability, sleep loss, mental fuzziness, and memory loss do happen. You may even feel depressed; but *major depression*, a big-time mental illness, does not especially plague perimenopausal women. As a matter of fact, there is less mental illness in the middle years than earlier in life, and you may find that sufficiently reassuring. Still, if you can't remember where you put the blasted car keys, and you find that *irritating*, then you would probably benefit from knowing why it happens and what you can do about it.

OK, SO WHY IS THIS HAPPENING?

Estrogen receptors exist in your brain, so the presence or absence of that hormone has a potent influence on the neurotransmission of brain impulses across synapses (connecting points between nerve cells). A variety of chemicals in the brain, called neurotransmitters, carry the impulses (messages) across each synapse. Estrogen loss not only diminishes the total number of synapses, but also decreases the level of the neurotransmitter chemicals. Since estrogen receptors are also in the part of your brain that governs emotions, it is not surprising that fluctuations in hormone levels can induce up-and-down emotional responses.

Withdrawal of this female hormone from your brain cells is not unlike the withdrawal of an addicting drug such as cocaine, nicotine, or tranquilizers. The cells with estrogen receptors are not getting their "fix" of estrogen. This triggers symptoms like moodiness, irritability, and anger until the number of receptors decreases sufficiently. In perimenopause, there may be a waxing and waning of effective estrogen, so that the receptors are at times supplied quite well and at other times left wanting. Eventually the receptors die off, but this can take one to two years and, occasionally, up to 10 years. A gradual diminution of estrogen results in milder symptoms, but a sudden withdrawal, as from quitting hormone replacement or having your ovaries removed surgically, may cause intense symptoms.

Emotional peaks and valleys are linked to all episodes of major hormonal change in women's lives, such as the ferment in the teens, and the dramatic hormone increases of pregnancy. It is hardly surprising that the hormonal disequilibrium of perimenopause should cause these emotional changes again.

SECONDARY EFFECTS OF ESTROGEN DEFICIENCY

Not all brain symptoms are directly related to hormone deficiency, but they can be caused by problems that *are* hormone related. For example, hot flashes and resulting sleep disruptions are definitely associated with estrogen deficiency. Hot flashes tend to decrease REM (rapid eye movement) sleep, the most beneficial type of sleep. Chronic sleep deprivation causes fatigue, irritability, headaches, and minor depression. As long ago as 1977, Campbell and Whitehead found that estrogen stopped hot flashes. Then a domino effect followed: with no hot flashes one benefitted from better sleep, which resulted in relief of fatigue, less irritability, fewer headaches, and relief of minor depression. Benefits were maximized if the hormones were taken at bedtime to get the highest blood level during the night. They also found that estrogen has a tonic effect on memory loss and anxiety and an overall beneficial effect on mood. If *testosterone*, the male hormone, is added to estrogen, there is further enhancement of this mental tonic effect. With both hormones, women feel more serene, more cheerful, and more energetic. Sexual desire improves too.

Certain life situations may contribute to perimenopausal symptoms. Raising teenagers who are coping with their own hormone upheaval can be gasoline on the fire for a perimenopausal woman. The same can be said for raising a small child. A loveless relationship, an impending divorce, or even a new relationship may all be very difficult to manage when you feel only marginally in control.

WELL THEN, WHAT CAN I DO ABOUT IT?

Control is a key word here. During this trying time, many negative emotions surface unbidden to dominate your thoughts and speech. A trivial incident causes utter outrage: "What do you *mean* you forgot the loaf of bread? You *never* remember anything I say. Why do you even come home if you hate me so much?" Heavy, right? Many women feel frazzled, discombobulated, and so otherwise distracted that short-term memory becomes a shambles. Car keys disappear, appointments are forgotten, and returning phone calls becomes a lost art. Perimenopausal women feel helpless to control these things; it's like trying to halt a runaway train. Many feel like an alien spirit has inhabited their body, and they are forced to stand aside and watch the carnage.

Herein lie some of the clues for dealing with these changes. Usually the extremes are not an all-day, every-day thing. They come and go, so when you are feeling yourself again, take time to reflect on your out-of-character responses. You will probably recognize that you were in one of your funks when it happened. Although you didn't or couldn't control it, you can at least recognize that it was indeed a funk. It can be very helpful to alert the people important to you when one of these moods is upon you. Let them know that it isn't intentional, that it will be temporary, and that it does not in any way imply that you do not love them. Ask that they leave you in peace as much as possible; put off conflicts until your equanimity has returned. Suggest that they make a written note of the potentially divisive issue, and defer the agenda for the time being . . . but not indefinitely. Maybe a day or two. You need to know, and those around you need to know, that your changed emotions are physiologic in origin (hormone disequilibrium) and not psychological. This is not lunacy; and you do not need to be taken off to "the home." This a fluctuating, day-to-day change that will not be permanent.

DEPRESSION

Depression is an important topic. This is one of the most overused, and misused, words in our culture. Depression has become part of the lexicon of all age groups: "I'm depressed because my mother didn't put Twinkies in my lunch bag"; "Studying for finals is depressing"; "It's depressing that my kids hate the neighbors." Disappointment or dissatisfaction more accurately describe the above examples; depression is very unlikely to be the case.

We commonly speak of depression in the same breath as menopause. Studies show that perimenopause does not *cause* depression, although depression may coexist in women who are perimenopausal (McKinlay 1987). Perimenopausal symptoms may aggravate an existing depression. These two situations share some common symptoms such as

- ✦ reduced sex drive and sexual responsiveness
- ✦ irritability
- ✦ mood instability
- ✦ decreased energy
- ✦ tearfulness
- ✦ interrupted sleep
- ✦ worry and anxiety
- ✦ emotional detachment

With this degree of commonality between perimenopausal symptoms and depression, it is obviously important to carefully distinguish which is causing what.

Major depression is a significant mental illness. It is now known to be caused by chemical imbalances of *serotonin* (a neurotransmitter) in your brain. It requires psychotherapy and, often, psychotherapeutic drugs such as Prozac. McKinlay's 1987 study showed that depression tends to occur more frequently in younger than midlife women. For women who are perimenopausal *and* depressed, HRT is not necessarily the answer. It may relieve some of the perimenopausal symptoms aggravating the depression, but it won't in any way improve a depression that has its roots in a poor relationship, occupational threats, financial crises, or other chronic stressors. The message, therefore, is to avoid simply accepting a prescription for hormones if you feel low. If HRT *is* started and your depression fails to improve, insist on a psychiatric consultation.

The other side of this coin is the woman whose perimenopausal cognitive symptoms have been misinterpreted by her doctor as anxiety or depression. A psychotherapeutic drug may be prescribed. In this situation, checking the FSH level may help to reveal the true state of affairs. Your doctor can then recommend the appropriate therapy. Estrogen therapy, when needed, can be magic.

It is helpful to understand the diagnostic criteria for major depression. Read over Table 3-2. If these criteria describe you accurately or even closely, I urge

---

Table 3-2

SYMPTOMS OF A MAJOR DEPRESSIVE EPISODE

Have you had at least five of the following symptoms during the same two week period? Is this a change from your usual functioning?

1. Depressed mood most of the day, nearly every day.
    or
2. Markedly diminished interest or pleasure in all, or almost all, activities most of the day, nearly everyday.
    and
3. Significant weight loss or weight gain even when not dieting (e.g., more than 5% of body weight in a month). Increased or decreased appetite nearly every day.
4. Insomnia or hypersomnia nearly every day.
5. Psychomotor agitation or retardation nearly every day.
6. Fatigue or loss of energy nearly every day.
7. Feelings of worthlessness. Excessive or inappropriate guilt nearly every day.
8. Diminished ability to think or concentrate, or indecisiveness nearly every day.
9. Recurrent thoughts of death (not just fear of dying), recurrent suicidal thoughts without a specific plan, a suicidal attempt, or a plan for suicide.

Yes answers to 1 or 2 *and* to any four items from 3–9 suggest you may have a major depression.

Source: *Diagnostic and Statistical Manual of Mental Disorders*, 3d ed. (1987)

you to seek a psychiatric consultation. Major depression is very treatable, but I must reemphasize that HRT is not the answer. Nor will HRT help psychological disturbances associated with relationship problems, occupational distress, or financial trouble.

Let's Do Something about Perimenopause

There are a ton of management regimens out there for dealing with perimenopause, some of them worthwhile, and some not. Most work for some people, but none works for all. They include diet, exercise, herbs, stress management, hormone replacement, biofeedback, acupuncture, yoga, meditation, prayer, quitting smoking, and other practices.

DESIGNING A PLAN

How do you find your way through a seeming blizzard of sometimes conflicting advice?

First, do what you are now doing: Educate yourself. Read this book and others. Look carefully at the credentials and qualifications of the writer. Look also at the motivations of the authors. Are they selling something? Are they trying to convert you to a certain belief? You will find some works that are subtly negative, and some that are slashingly critical of others' beliefs. On the other hand, some writers are much too casual and treat this midlife transition so lightly as to appear cavalier in their approach. Don't forget lectures, seminars, video and audio tapes, focus groups, and educational TV programs.

Second, talk to your doctor about your concerns. Evaluate your physician's interest in and knowledge of perimenopause and menopause. Then, if you are comfortable, formulate a game plan for current and future management. If you know what to expect as your transition progresses, you will be less dismayed or confused when confronted with the myriad problems that may lie ahead—or greatly pleased if they don't ever happen. Actual management plans will likely revolve around hormone replacement, stress management, proper nutrition, and an exercise program.

Third, evaluate alternative medical care plans. Most physicians, like me, have been trained in "Western" medical disciplines; but others exist, and their validity, as well as effectiveness, is becoming more widely recognized. Homeopathy, Chinese herbal medicine, acupuncture, and holistic medicine are a few examples, and they are covered in Chapter 12.

Mind/body medicine is being seriously explored by talented people who have reported stunning successes in dealing with a variety of ailments. The future appears fascinating for this field, which bases itself on the tenet that healing derives from our own inner selves and from the power of our minds to influence disordered bodily functioning. I urge you to read *Quantum Healing*, written by Deepak Chopra, M.D. Dr. Chopra, an endocrinologist (hormone specialist), writes clearly and honestly about mind/body medicine and does not hesitate to point out that results have been hard to interpret to date. There has been great interest for several years in mind/body techniques such as biofeedback, behavior modification, hypnotism, visualization, transcendental meditation, and others. Like most medical regimens, universal success is elusive. Nevertheless, mind/body medicine is emerging as a field, rather than a concept. As reliability improves, future successes may be mind-boggling.

HORMONE TREATMENT DILEMMAS

Dealing with the symptoms of perimenopause can be frustrating because there commonly is waxing and waning of estrogen production. This can make taking estrogen supplements alternatively effective and useless. Furthermore, symptoms may have multiple sources. Hot flashes are an early symptom, but not all are due to estrogen depletion. Indeed, about 25% of women in their reproductive years have occasional hot flashes that are *not* relieved by hormone therapy. Menstrual cycle changes and mood swings can have other causes. Whether or not a hormone regimen should be offered is often a troublesome issue.

The current feeling of leaders in this field is that a trial of hormone supplements is justified if you are having typical symptoms of estrogen deficiency and they are occurring within the typical age range. Table 3-3 lists the symptoms you could experience. No one has all of these estrogen deficiency effects, thank heavens, but any combination of them may make an appearance. Figure 3-1 shows you an approximate age at which some of the symptoms may be expected to occur. With this information, you and your doctor can arrive at a decision as to whether or not a hormone supplement is reasonable for you. It would be handy to be able to rely on simple laboratory tests for guidance, but rising and falling levels of estrogen production during perimenopause makes this impractical and expensive. In recent years the most frequently utilized method of perimenopausal hormone supplementation has been the low dose birth control pill. There are many advantages to this including symptom control as well as prevention of pregnancy. This will be more thoroughly covered in Chapter 11.

Table 3-3
SYMPTOMS AND SIGNS OF ESTROGEN LOSS

Irregular periods
Hot flashes
Mood swings
Fragmented sleep
Short-term memory loss
Difficulty concentrating
Irritability
Anxiety
Minor depression
Skin dryness
Wrinkling
Reduced sexual lubrication
Vaginal dryness
Decreased sexual desire
Reduced muscle tone
Reduced stamina
Constipation
Recurrent urinary tract infection
Breast sagging
Eye dryness
Underactive thyroid
Osteoporosis
Rise in cholesterol
Beginning risk of heart disease

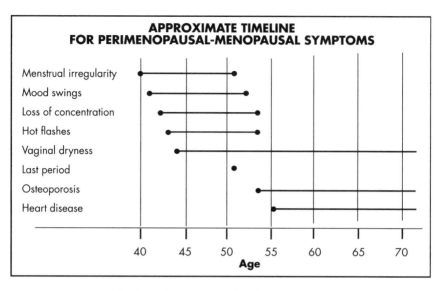

**APPROXIMATE TIMELINE
FOR PERIMENOPAUSAL-MENOPAUSAL SYMPTOMS**

Menstrual irregularity	
Mood swings	
Loss of concentration	
Hot flashes	
Vaginal dryness	
Last period	
Osteoporosis	
Heart disease	

Age: 40   45   50   55   60   65   70

If hormone use *is* indicated, and if you decide to start it, then some dramatic changes will take place. Hot flashes will disappear in a week to a month. Menstrual irregularities will get straightened out in a few cycles, depending on the type of hormone regimen used (there are several). A feeling of well-being will replace your moodiness. Short-term memory will improve (the car keys will start showing up where they're supposed to be). With control of hot flashes, you will sleep better; fatigue will disappear, and other cognitive changes will improve. You will feel like a whole woman again, and those closest to you will be well aware of this change. I do not mean for this to sound like estrogen replacement is some magic elixir that you merely swallow and . . . Bingo! . . . it's the new you. The improvement is gradual and is often only realized when you think to compare the previous few weeks with now.

If a trial of taking hormone supplements consistently improves your symptoms, you can proceed to long-term hormone replacement and other preventive measures with confidence. Other nonhormonal methods of symptom control are available, however, and you will learn more about them in Section III. Whether you decide on traditional medical care or alternative care is absolutely your call. You make the choice based on your own beliefs, knowledge, and expectations.

Men Can Help . . . Really

Your man really *can* help, but, like you, he needs to know what is going on before trying to do something about it. Much of the time, your problem with him, if you have one, can be greatly improved if he makes the effort to become informed about female climacteric (menopause-related) changes. Armed with information, he will better understand what is happening in your body and your mind. The two of you will then be more likely to discuss all of this in a milieu of cooperation and understanding.

In his book *Men Are From Mars, Women Are From Venus*, psychologist John Gray points out that one of the fundamental differences between women and men is in their approach to handling a problem. A woman finds satisfaction in simply being able to discuss a problem with someone who gives her their attention and sympathetic understanding. On the other hand, a man needs to deal with a problem by solving it. Discussion, while enlightening, is not enough for men.

Take this scenario as an example. You come home tired and frazzled; your hot flashes have been disrupting your sleep so much that you are chronically fatigued. The company you work for is downsizing. They are getting rid of many workers your age, and you can only stay competitive in keeping your job by taking on more responsibility. What you want to hear from him is: "Well *sweetheart*, no *wonder* you're so tired. Sit down and relax while I fix you something to drink; and we'll talk about it." But instead, "Mr. Problem Solver" goes into his Force-Four Fix-it mode and says: "Just quit that lousy job. They have never treated you right, and they're getting worse. So tell 'em to shove it . . . *Next* problem please."

We are very unlikely to change our differing ways of dealing with problems, *because that is just the way women are and the way men are.* If you and your partner are to get along however, each needs to understand how the other one works and to make every effort to respond to a problem in a fashion that accommodates the partner's needs.

So tell your man that you would very much appreciate his reading this book, or at least Chapter 17 entitled "Just For Men: Andropause and Menopause." He can also read other books, listen to tapes, or attend seminars and lectures with you. Let him know that he does not have to solve all of your problems. Some of them are yours alone, so don't burden his inborn problem-solving urge with something that will frustrate him and put the two of you on different pages. But he *can* help . . . really.

Summing Up

This chapter has painted a fairly grim picture of what may happen to you during perimenopause. Please realize that none of these things may occur to you. Those symptoms that do surface may not be bothersome for you. Long-term studies uniformly indicate that 80% of women experience perimenopause without significant difficulty and regard it as a normal physiologic event in their lives. Also realize that effective help is available if you need it. Perimenopause is a transition to the fuller life that awaits you. So be of good cheer, and continue your education about this phase of your life.

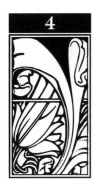

PERIMENOPAUSAL PREGNANCY
YES, IT CAN HAPPEN

Yogi Berra was referring to baseball games when he said, "It ain't over till it's over," but he could just as well have been talking about fecundity. Fecundity is doctor-speak for fruitfulness, or fertility. Your fecundity, or ability to successfully reproduce, gradually declines starting in your early 30s. By the time you are in your 40s, fecundity is on a real downhill roll. Many perimenopausal conceptions never progress beyond a few days or a few weeks of pregnancy before a spontaneous abortion (miscarriage) occurs. Clinically recognized spontaneous abortion occurs in only 12% of women under age 20, but in women over 40, the rate is 26%.

If You Want to Get Pregnant

The proportion of births in women aged 35 to 49 is expected to rise from 5% in 1982 to 8.6% by 2000, an increase of 72%. Perimenopausal pregnancies are becoming more common because so many women are delaying marriage and then establishing a career before considering a family. Perimenopausal women considering pregnancy are confronted with two major concerns: the increased rate of complications associated with pregnancy in midlife, and the increased difficulty of achieving a pregnancy. The highest risks for pregnancy complications are in the early part of the reproductive era (teens) and the latter part of the era (40s).

Pregnancy after 35, and especially after 40, is fraught with greater risk for chromosomal abnormalities in the fetus such as Down syndrome and neural tube defects involving the brain and spinal cord. This is related to the fact that conception with an older egg represents an increased risk of a faulty chromosome exchange with sperm chromosomes. Fortunately, testing for these chromosome defects is readily available and reliable. Amniocentesis (the collection of fluid from inside the uterus) and chorionic villus sampling (the collection of placental tissue cells) are both tests that can be done early in pregnancy to evaluate whether the baby has a normal chromosome compliment. The newer *triple marker testing* is based on three maternal blood tests for *alpha-fetoprotein* (AFP), *human chorionic gonadotropin* (hCG), and *unconjugated estriol*. The blood tests do not make the diagnosis of fetal defects, but they are a means of providing a percentage likelihood for a fetal problem. If it appears that the risk for Down syndrome or a neural tube defect is high, ultrasound examination of the fetus can be done. Also the more invasive, and therefore more risky, amniocentesis and chorionic villus sampling can be carried out for a more reliable diagnosis.

A 1993 study by Drs. Vicki Edge and Russell Laros found that there is no increased risk in perimenopausal pregnancy for chronic diseases such as heart disease, high blood pressure, diabetes, or lupus. There was, however, greater risk for pregnancy induced problems like preeclampsia (pregnancy induced hypertension), fibroid growth, pregnancy induced diabetes, fetal distress in labor, and abnormal labor patterns. Because of these problems, the cesarean section rate is higher than in younger women. Nevertheless, Edge and Laros found that the babies borne by perimenopausal women were just as healthy as in younger women.

If you are planning a perimenopausal pregnancy, get a good health check first and correct any problems that may exist. A healthy lifestyle is very important to your being successful, so good nutrition and adequate regular exercise are essential. The following are additional precautions:

+ if you are diabetic, your disease must be under good control prior to conception
+ take folic acid 0.4 mg daily prior to conception to reduce the risk of neural tube defects
+ stop birth control pills several months before pregnancy. The pill causes your endometrium to become thin which jeopardizes implantation of a newly fertilized egg
+ stop alcohol, tobacco, and recreational drugs. All of them increase the risk of pregnancy loss and fetal damage
+ vaccinations for measles, mumps, rubella (German measles), and hepatitis B should be current
+ clear up any sexually transmitted diseases. They can affect your ability to get pregnant and can infect your baby

- if you have AIDS, you must be on the antiviral drug AZT. It reduces the chance of your baby getting the disease from 33% to 8%
- get under care as soon as you know you have become pregnant. It is better to have had prepregnancy care

If You Can't

Infertility is increasingly common after 40. It is based on a number of factors common to this age range:

- ovulation is less reliable and therefore less frequent
- sexual frequency is diminished for most couples
- sperm count and sperm motility are lower in older partners
- obstructive tubal disease from sexually transmitted diseases is more common if you have had multiple partners
- Pituitary dysfunction may be a factor with abnormal production of FSH, LH, TSH (thyroid stimulating hormone), and prolactin. Normal production of all these hormones is necessary to successfully become pregnant

Fertility drugs such as clomiphene citrate and gonadotropins can be helpful to women who have hormonal infertility. The pregnancy rate is not high with these methods, but they increase the chances for success. For others, *assisted reproductive technologies* (ART) can be the answer. These are the so-called test-tube pregnancies. They involve fertilizing an egg with sperm under laboratory conditions. Sometimes a donor egg is used. The successful pregnancy rate is not high with these techniques either, but many couples are helped by them.

If You Don't Want To

For those of you who are not intending a pregnancy, the take home message is that you cannot depend on perimenopause to protect you from an unplanned pregnancy. So, we better discuss what will.

The best policy is to use contraception until one year after your final menstrual period or until your LH (luteinizing hormone from the pituitary) rises and stays up. This indicates that your ovaries are not capable of ovulating. The contraception menu is really quite extensive:

✦ *Abstinence.* It works fine, but it's a bummer for most.

✦ *Barrier methods.* Latex (male and female) condoms are especially important to use if you are not in a mutually monogamous relationship. This is true even if you are postmenopausal. They have been shown to reduce the incidence of sexually transmitted disease (STD), which holds no respect for age. If you are having painful sex, condoms may aggravate it unless you use plenty of lubricant. Be sure to avoid Vaseline, since petroleum jelly weakens latex. Use a vaginal spermicide containing nonoxynol-9 in addition to condoms for additional contraceptive protection. The female condom was marketed a few years ago amid great expectations because it was the first STD protector that was woman-controlled. Unfortunately is has a high failure rate in pregnancy protection; so it is unlikely that it will be available much longer. Some aging men experience inadequate erection with condoms because they require more direct penile stimulation, which condoms may diminish. In that case the diaphragm with a spermicide is an effective contraceptive, but of little help in STD prevention.

✦ *Intrauterine device (IUD).* This is a very effective method, which may be especially useful for perimenopausal women. There are only two on the market in the United States. The Copper T 380-A, or ParaGard, can stay in place for 10 years and span the entire climacteric era. It is important that you have a mutually monogamous relationship, since outside partners increase the risk of pelvic infection with an IUD in the uterus. The other IUD is the Progestasert, a progesterone containing device that works well but must be replaced annually. A new progesterone-containing IUD from Finland is now being tested. When it finally gets through all the FDA hoops, this IUD will be good for seven years.

✦ *Norplant.* This relatively recent method utilizes progestin (synthetic progesterone) contained in six silastic capsules that are implanted under the skin of the upper inner arm. It can remain in place for five years. The failure rate is 0.2% in the first year, which rises to 1.6% by the fourth year and then drops again to 0.4%. Progestin may cause minor depression in some women. Irregular bleeding is common in the first one to two years and may be especially perplexing for perimenopausal women. It requires a minor surgical office procedure for implantation and for removal. Removal has been a problem for some, and Norplant is currently being assaulted by the class action law suit culture, although it has a good record of safety and effectiveness. The makers of Norplant are working on using only two pellets which will be easier to insert and to remove. Biodegradable pellets may solve removal problems in the future.

◆ *Depo-Provera (DMPA).* A long acting progestin called *depo-medroxy-progesterone acetate*, or *DMPA*, is given by injection every three months. At 0.1% to 0.7%, it has a very low failure rate. As well as offering effective contraception, it helps prevent endometrial cancer. In fact, for many years and until recently, its only FDA-approved use was for treatment of endometrial cancer. Now, a growing number of physicians are prescribing it for contraceptive use. Like with other progestins, some women will feel depressed. Irregular bleeding can be a problem. This method may result in infertility for some women for up to nine months after the last injection; but it is not permanent. The question has been raised that there may be an increased risk of breast cancer in young women who use this method for over 36 months. Three studies, in Costa Rica, New Zealand, and by the World Health Organization, have produced conflicting results. Their validity was hampered by the small number of women studied, according to the ACOG Committee Opinion #135 of April 1994.

◆ *Morning after pill.* This can be useful if you have had unprotected sex about the time of ovulation. It must be used within 72 hours of having sex and has an effectiveness of about 98%–99%. Two tablets of Ovral or another equivalent dose birth control pill should be taken and repeated 12 hours later. Premarin (conjugated estrogen) in a high dose taken three times daily for five days also works well but is fraught with nausea for many women. If you are perimenopausal and your cycles are irregular, a problem with this method can be the uncertainty as to whether or not you were near ovulation at the time of unprotected sex.

◆ *RU-486.* This French medication has been used successfully to abort a proven early pregnancy. RU-486 blocks progesterone production by the ovaries and will prevent implantation of a fertilized ovum, so it works like the morning after pill. It has not been licensed for use in the United States, but in July 1996 the FDA medical advisory committee recommended that French results of clinical trials be accepted, so it may be approved in the future.

◆ *Rhythm method (timed abstinence).* This method is based on knowing when you will ovulate and avoiding sex two days before and two days after egg release. This method is fraught with many miscalculations, especially for perimenopausal women because their cycles are no longer rhythmic. The failure rate for all ages is 48%, although for women over 40, who are less fertile and may have less frequent sex, the failure rate is considerably lower.

◆ *Tubal sterilization.* In this out-patient surgical operation usually performed through two or three Band-Aid–size incisions in the abdomen, a laparoscope (a tube allowing internal visual examination) and other instruments are inserted to interrupt the fallopian tubes. This prevents sperm from getting upstream and eggs from getting downstream. It works well (two in 100 women may later get pregnant); but it should be regarded as permanent, and it *is* surgery. A reversal operation is technically possible, but the success rate is discouraging. Side effects are not common but can include altered ovarian function from local surgical trauma, which may shorten ovarian life. Tubal ligation lowers the subsequent risk for ovarian cancer by 67% because it eliminates carcinogens that enter your pelvis by migration upward from your vagina.

✦ *Vasectomy.* An effective male sterilization operation done with local anesthesia in the office, it should be regarded as permanent. A reversal procedure is possible, but expensive and not always effective. When a vasectomy has been several years in the past, antibodies sometimes form which attach to the sperm cells and render them ineffective. In this situation, vasectomy reversal would not be indicated. Some men emotionally equate vasectomy with castration. Even though it does not eliminate male hormone production, a few men will have long-term sexual dysfunction anyhow. Careful and thoughtful counseling beforehand will avoid this for most.

✦ *Low dose birth control pills.* Low dose pills are very effective for perimenopausal women. They can be used right up to menopause in low risk candidates, meaning nonsmokers. This method combines both estrogen and progestin which effectively controls perimenopausal symptoms including menstrual irregularity, hot flashes, and mood swings. The pill also helps maintain bone density, protects against heart disease, and reduces the risk of endometrial and ovarian cancer. It helps protect against benign breast disease, rheumatoid arthritis, benign ovarian cysts, anemia, and pelvic inflammatory disease. In addition, a 1996 study by Darney showed that perimenopausal women who were on the pill for 10 years have a 600% decrease in heart attacks. The protection lasts for 15 years after stopping the pill. The study also showed that after 10 years of pill use, the rate of ovarian cancer was reduced by 85%, uterine cancer was down by 50%, and breast cancer by 35%. The low dose combination pill can make for really smooth sailing during perimenopause. When menopause has occurred, signaled by estrogen deficiency symptoms during the week in the cycle you're off hormones, you can switch over to standard HRT, if that is your choice. The standard estrogen dosage in HRT is about 75% lower than the low dose pill.

✦ *Progestin-only pill (mini-pill).* The mini-pill contains no estrogen. It is an effective contraceptive which must be taken on a daily basis, 365 days per year. Its use may be initially fraught with irregular bleeding,

Table 4-1
UNPLANNED PREGNANCY RATE FOR WOMEN
Age 35–44

Tubal ligation	1.8%
IUD	1.7%
Birth control pill	1.9%
Condom	3.3%
Rhythm method	6.2%
Spermicides	9.1%
Diaphragm & cervical cap	10.3%

but bleeding sometimes stops altogether in perimenopausal women. Progestin helps protect against endometrial cancer as well as loss of bone density, though not as well as estrogen. There is some benefit in controlling hot flashes. The mini-pill can be a good choice for perimenopausal women who cannot, or must not, take estrogen. It may help your contraceptive planning to know the relative effectiveness of many of the above methods. Table 4-1 lists them in order of protectiveness.

Since the 1970s, the appearance of new contraceptive methods in the United States has slowed to a glacial pace. Political posturing, bureaucratic regulation, and liability concerns have all played a role in slowing research. European and other industrialized countries have all benefited much more from new devices and techniques than the United States has. Nevertheless, significant research is under way and new methods are on the horizon:

✦ *Spermicides* are being developed that are stronger and will inhibit HIV, chlamydia, trichomonads, and other infectious agents from multiplying in your vagina or from adhering to vaginal walls. They are being tested in new disposable diaphragms.

✦ *Injectables* that last six to eight months, as compared to Depo Provera which lasts three months, are being investigated.

✦ *Biodegradable implants* using only two capsules are coming. Norplant uses six silastic capsules that must be surgically removed after five years.

✦ *Biodegradable pellets* containing progestin are being developed. They are about the size of a rice kernel, can be injected under the skin, and will dissolve after two years. A similar method using a biodegradable microcapsule containing a time-release hormone will be injected and provide contraception for one to six months.

✦ *Progestin gel* may be available to rub into the skin.

✦ *Vaginal rings* impregnated with estrogen and progestin, or progestin alone, are being used in Europe. An estrogen-containing ring, called Estring, became available in the United States in February 1997. It is being used for women who have atrophic (thinning) changes in vaginal and bladder lining tissues, but not for contraception. The ring is about the size of a diaphragm, but is hollow. It can be left in place during sex or removed briefly without loss of effectiveness.

✦ *Contraceptive vaccines* that would immunize against the pregnancy hormone hCG (*human chorionic gonadotropin*), which is necessary in the first trimester to maintain pregnancy, are being researched. Vaccines may also be developed to attack sperm or to oppose a fertilized egg.

Many of you reading this book may not need any of these newer methods by the time they have filtered their way through the serpentine and time consuming paths required for new products. But at least you know that they may be on the way.

Summing Up

Perimenopausal pregnancy can be a problem both from the standpoint of its being unintended and that it may be difficult to achieve. Adequate measures exist to successfully accomplish both goals. Diminished pregnancy concerns relieve a major source of anxiety for perimenopausal women. Your transition will be so much smoother if you get a handle on it.

SECTION II

MENOPAUSE

By definition, menopause is simply that point in time when you have your last menstrual period. There are no more periods; they are over, finished, through, and done. In the climacteric years, menopause is the dividing line between perimenopause and postmenopause. This section of the book has been entitled "Menopause," but it is really about postmenopause too, since it covers certain conditions and events that become noticeable *after* your final menstrual period. Menopause is the commonly used term for this era, however, so that's what we'll go with. I'm not trying to change the world here.

No More Periods? Why Should I Worry?

Menopause, at age 51, is a natural event in the aging process. That it is natural is comforting, but the catch is that the withdrawal of female hormones from your body is actually *harmful* to you. It accelerates the aging process of certain parts of your body: heart, blood vessels, bone, skin, vagina, bladder, urethra, and brain. Well then:

Q: Is it natural or not? A: Yes it is.
Q: Can I prevent it? A: Nope.
Q: Is it risky? A: Yep.
Q: Can I alter the risks in my favor? A: You bet.

Section II will first cover the low profile, nontransitory, and serious threats that can indeed shorten your life. These include heart disease, osteoporosis, and cancer. Next will be discussed the nonlethal but unwelcome bodily changes to your skin, breasts, and vagina that constitute strikes at highly regarded feminine features. Midlife sex for women and for men is in this section as well. Prevention and treatment options for the various problems will be discussed.

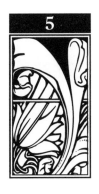

CARDIOVASCULAR DISEASE
THE 900-POUND GORILLA

Cardiovascular disease (CVD) is the most serious and most ominous of all postmenopausal problems. This chapter will show you the magnitude of the threat that CVD poses for you. You will learn the roles of low-density lipoprotein (LDL) and high-density lipoprotein (HDL) in causing CVD. Estrogen's overpowering influence in preventing CVD is detailed, as well as the downside aspects of estrogen use. Lifestyle changes that are necessary to maintain cardiovascular health will be discussed.

Let's Look at Some Numbers

Cardiovascular disease means heart and blood vessel disease. In the United States, CVD is the leading cause of death for postmenopausal women. The lifetime risk for developing CVD is two out of three women, and the lifetime probability for a woman of dying of a heart attack is 31%. It is not only the number one cause of death for women, it is also the major cause of disability in older women. Table 5-1 illustrates the magnitude of this threat.

Just *look* at those numbers. Heart attack death is five times more frequent than breast cancer death. Other studies have indicated that heart attack death is as much as 10 times more frequent than breast cancer death. Did you know that? Have the headlines convinced you that breast cancer is the number one problem you face? Heart attack is also 10 times more likely than the combined deaths from cancer of all reproductive organs: cervix, uterus, and ovaries. It is

Table 5-1	
DEATH RATES IN AMERICAN WOMEN	
Condition	Annual deaths per 100,000 women age 50–75
Coronary heart disease	10,500
Breast cancer	1,875
Osteoporotic bone fracture	938
Endometrial (uterine lining) cancer	188

Adapted from Henderson and others, *American Journal of Obstetrics & Gynecology* 154:1181 (1986)

10 times more likely than osteoporosis death, and 50 times that of uterine cancer death. In the 1990s, more women are dying from heart attacks than men are. For postmenopausal women, CVD is indeed the 900-pound gorilla. You can *not* ignore it.

THAT SOUNDS AWFUL. WHAT ARE MY CHANCES?

Your chances of developing heart disease are influenced by a number of factors. Some of them are just the cards you have been dealt genetically; some of them are fully in your control to alter favorably. Look at the following list of risk factors and see if any of these apply to you:

+ close relatives (parent or sibling) who died of heart disease before age 60. There's nothing you can do about that situation except turn it into a wakeup call for your own prevention program
+ diabetic. This raises your risk of CVD dramatically
+ postmenopausal and not on HRT. More on this below
+ personal history of unexplained chest pain
+ smoke cigarettes. Increases your risk four times over that of nonsmokers. If you quit, your risk remains high for two years, but after four years the risk is no higher than those who have never smoked
+ weigh 20% or more above ideal level. Mild to moderate obesity more than doubles your risk
+ have high blood pressure, more than 140/90
+ have high cholesterol. More on this below
+ lead a sedentary lifestyle. Physically active women have a 60%–75% lower risk than those who are inactive

Once you have a heart attack, you are twice as likely to die from it as men are. This may be because women are generally older than men when heart attacks occur, and other health problems may also be present which complicate treatment. In addition, many physicians are not as alert to the female symptoms of heart attack because of past bias that it is a "male" problem. *Coronary bypass surgery* was developed for the male heart, and twice as many women fail to survive it as men. This is partly because you have a smaller heart with smaller blood vessels, which are more difficult to deal with surgically. Another additive factor can be that delayed recognition of your symptoms may have delayed your bypass, and you are sicker as well as older when the operation is undertaken. The same is true for coronary *angioplasty*, the "roto-rooter" operation where a catheter with a balloon attachment is used to flatten the obstruction in the artery. The instruments were designed for larger male arteries. As a result, there is greater difficulty, more complications with torn vessels, and a survival rate reduced by half for women.

These data make a bitter pill to swallow, but they will improve as health care professionals become reeducated about female CVD and as you yourself become proactive regarding prevention of the serious threat that CVD poses for you. So educate yourself about a heart-healthy lifestyle and especially about your ace in the hole: estrogen.

Estrogen to the Rescue

For coronary heart disease, the death rate is reduced by over 50% if estrogen is used after menopause. Several major health studies, using statistically significant numbers of women, have shown this (Speroff 1994). The Nurses' Health Study surveyed 121,964 women of whom 32,317 were post-menopausal (Stampfer 1985). The study showed a 50% reduction of coronary heart disease in those who had ever used estrogen, and a 70% reduction if they were currently using it. Similar results came from the Lipid Research Clinics Follow-Up Study with a 63% decrease in deaths from heart disease for current estrogen users (Bush 1987). Another 1986 study by Henderson and others amazingly showed a 16% decrease in deaths from *all* causes for estrogen users.

More recently, researchers at the University of Southern California reported in 1991 that the decrease in overall death rate was greater, the longer the estrogen was taken. Users of 15 years duration had 40% fewer deaths from any cause than nonusers.

Part of the reason that heart disease has been regarded as essentially a male problem by most people, the medical field included, is that women are protected from it during the childbearing years by estrogen. After menopause and estrogen decline, women start getting more heart disease, although they continue to lag behind men for about 10 years. By age 60–70, however, about 50% of female deaths are from heart disease, just as in men. The big point here is that it does not have to be that way for you. Estrogen is cardioprotective, and this fact is not controversial. The evidence is not ambiguous. Estrogen protects your heart, and this is the most significant life benefit that it offers you for a disease that outranks breast cancer deaths fivefold and osteoporosis tenfold.

HOW CAN ONE HORMONE DO ALL THAT?

I will try to be simple and brief in a rather technical explanation. The protection comes from the positive effect of estrogen on *lipoprotein* blood levels. *Lipid* refers to fat; lipoproteins are fat and protein combined and function as cholesterol carriers in your bloodstream. Cholesterol is a waxy substance that has a variety of vital bodily uses, but it is not in itself a fat. The two most important lipoproteins are *low-density lipoprotein* (LDL) and *high-density lipoprotein* (HDL). The LDL cholesterol carrier is the black-hat bad guy that deposits cholesterol on blood vessel walls, causing narrowing of the vessels. This leads to high blood pressure, heart attacks, and strokes. HDL is the white-hat good guy that carries cholesterol back to your liver where is it

Table 5-2	
LIPID VALUES	
Total cholesterol	
Below 200 mg/ml	Desirable
200–240	At risk
Over 240	High risk
HDL cholesterol	
Above 50 mg/ml	Desirable
35–50	Good
Below 35	At risk
LDL cholesterol	
Below 130 mg/ml	Desirable
130–160	At risk
Above 160	High risk
Triglycerides	
Below 200 mg/ml	Normal
200–400	Borderline
400–1000	High
Above 1000	Very high
Cholesterol/HDL ratio	
Below 4.5	Desirable
Above 4.5	At risk

Source: National Cholesterol Education Program

excreted in bile. It may even remove LDL deposits from vessel walls. Well guess what folks? Estrogen raises your HDL and *lowers* your LDL!! More white hats than black hats, and that's good for our side.

Triglycerides are another lipid (fat) risk for you. They are a form of fatty acid that your body uses for energy or stores as body fat for later use. The liver makes some of them but most are derived from food. High triglycerides are a gender-specific risk factor because they play a greater role in CVD in women than in men. High levels combined with low HDL levels are a reliable predictor of heart disease in postmenopausal women. Studies have shown that high triglycerides in women are even a more important predictive factor for heart disease than your cholesterol level. Table 5-2 shows the target range for blood lipid values.

IT'S GOOD FOR YOU AND THE COUNTRY TOO

If you consider that the death rate from CVD in postmenopausal women is reduced by 50%–60% in estrogen users and that there are currently 46 million women in that category with 38 million boomers right on their heels, then the public health impact of this hormone is absolutely enormous. It is a simple fact that estrogen has the potential, when used properly, to prevent a lot of premature deaths and disability.

THAT WAS THE GOOD NEWS . . . ESTROGEN ISN'T PERFECT

I have thrust a lot of estrogen good news at you, and now I must temper it with some doubt, or some unknowns. I will explain more fully in Chapter 7 that estrogen, when used alone, increases the risk of endometrial (uterine lining) cancer. Progestin (synthetic version of progesterone), when combined with estrogen, reduces that cancer risk to the same level as nonusers of estrogen, so the current wisdom is to use the two of them together. But progestin is an *anti*-estrogen, which means it counteracts estrogen and reduces its beneficial effects. It does not *cancel* the benefits, as some poorly informed writers on this topic suggest, but it diminishes them slightly. The extent of the alteration is as follows: estrogen used alone increases HDL (the good guy) by about 12% and reduces LDL (the bad guy) by about 8%. When combined with progestin, the HDL only goes up about 6%, while LDL remains unchanged (Speroff 1994). Even this small negative effect diminishes with time. The findings of a University of Michigan study of more than 5,000 women were even more positive. The study found no significant difference between the HDL and LDL levels of those who used estrogen alone and those who used estrogen combined with progesterone. It was concluded that the risk of coronary heart disease is reduced by 40% in both groups.

The Women's Health Initiative (WHI), funded by the National Institutes of Health, is conducting studies to confirm or refute an adverse progestin effect. WHI is the largest prevention-of-disease study ever undertaken. It is a massive, prospective study to evaluate estrogen's influence on heart disease, osteoporosis, and breast cancer. When finished, in about the year 2005, scientists will know these answers with certainty. Another brief study of three years duration concluded that the favorable ratio of HDL exceeding LDL was maintained when progestin and estrogen were used together (Ravnikar 1989). That's great; but more confirmation with large, long-term studies like WHI is needed to really nail it down. So far, it looks like the progestin-estrogen combination will not result in a significant negative effect on the cardioprotective benefit of estrogen.

Dr. Leon Speroff, chairman of Ob/Gyn at Oregon Health Sciences University, is an internationally recognized expert in this field. He feels that, since the negative progestin effect is not more than a minimal decrease in HDL, then the risk of diminished cardiac protection will be quite small. Since convincing proof of this may still be several years away, and since the many benefits of estrogen are so important to women (see summary below), most physicians do not feel justified in withholding this hormone combination from their patients.

NOW SOME MORE GOOD NEWS

Speroff has summarized the cardiovascular benefits of estrogen better than anyone else in the field:

+ estrogen decreases your overall cholesterol blood level, and it lowers LDL cholesterol while raising HDL cholesterol (All winners)
+ estrogen prevents plaque formation in arteries (cholesterol deposits on the walls) that causes narrowing and leads to heart attacks and strokes. A monkey study in 1993 reported that estrogen actually *decreased* blood vessel wall deposits. This research study used estrogen and progesterone in combination (Clarkson 1993)
+ estrogen increases dilation of blood vessels, which improves flow of blood and lowers blood pressure
+ estrogen increases antiplatelet aggregation factors, which means it reduces the risk of blood clots that can cause heart attacks and strokes
+ estrogen has a direct strengthening effect on heart muscle, called an *inotropic* effect in doctor-speak, which results in more efficient heart action. This means more blood pumped per heartbeat
+ estrogen improves proper metabolism of glucose (sugar), so that less insulin is needed in your circulation. Too much circulating insulin causes big-time hardening of the arteries

♦ estrogen inhibits the usual postmenopausal accumulation of central abdominal fat, which is associated with hardening of the arteries

♦ estrogen is an antioxidant. It prevents oxidation of LDL, so it will not get deposited on the walls of blood vessels, causing hardening of the arteries (Speroff, 1994)

That is a pretty wide ranging list of benefits that estrogen provides for your cardiovascular system. It doesn't stop there, however. As you will see later in the book, estrogen has a positive influence on nearly any bodily tissue you can name. For now, we will stick to those effects relevant to CVD.

Antioxidants and Heart Disease

Basic research has suggested that antioxidant substances will lower the rate of coronary heart disease. They achieve this by preventing the oxidation of LDL so that it cannot be deposited as plaque on the walls of arteries. Estrogen has this effect, as discussed above, but there are other antioxidants that are also attracting interest. Vitamin E, beta-carotenes, and vitamin C are all naturally occurring antioxidants that have been studied. Researchers have reported significant decreases in coronary disease risk factors when a diet rich in antioxidant foods and supplements was used.

Vitamin E was the most beneficial in three large studies, with risk reductions ranging from 34%–46%. Beta-carotene was less helpful, averaging 26% reduction. Vitamin C, with an 18% average, was least influential. Other studies showed sharp variations from these results, and this muddied the creek for all except the vitamin industry. They jumped all over the positive information, and store shelves plus TV screens became loaded with vitamin supplements.

Others are now having a second look at the results of these early studies. They are questioning whether or not the research methods were sufficiently valid to justify recommending antioxidant supplements. An analysis by Harvard researchers Dr. Kathryn Rexrode and Dr. JoAnn Manson, published in a 1996 issue of *Menopausal Medicine*, commented that the studies receiving the most attention about antioxidants were based on the *cohort* method of analysis. This is a study technique in which a group of similar people (i.e., sharing certain factors, such as age, gender, and lifestyle, pertinent to the study) are observed over a period of time while they are tested for risk factors for a certain disease. In this particular case, the relation between heart disease and intake of antioxidants was studied. The problem with the cohort method is that of the people studied those who had the highest antioxidant intake of vitamin E, beta-carotene, and vitamin C were also the most likely to eat more fruits and vegetables, exercise more frequently, be more lean, and have other healthier lifestyle habits. This introduces doubt as to which lifestyle factors have been the most influential in achieving the positive results of lowered CVD risk factors.

A better scientific method is to use a *randomized clinical trial* in which a group of similar people (i.e., sharing certain factors, such as age, gender, and lifestyle, pertinent to the study) are studied over a period of time while using a prescribed diet or prescribed antioxidant supplements. The trial is randomized by putting some on the prescribed regimen and others not. Rexrode and Manson cited a few large-scale clinical trials that have been completed on beta-carotene that failed to find any benefit on CVD prevention. One study (the Beta-carotene and Retinol Efficacy Trials) on smokers using beta-carotene and vitamin A showed an increase in lung cancer. Another clinical study of vitamin E found only minor reductions in CVD mortality. No large-scale trials for vitamin C have been conducted. Ongoing clinical trials will provide additional future evidence of the value of antioxidant supplements, so keep tuned. Meanwhile Rexrode and Manson do not recommend antioxidant supplements. They do, however, recommend *dietary* intake of antioxidant vitamins. This seems a prudent course. See Table 5-3 for major food sources of these vitamins.

In contrast to the above study, in the May 2, 1996 issue of the *New England Journal of Medicine*, Dr. Walter Willett published the results of a study on women with proven heart disease. It was another vitamin E study. He found that an adequate intake of vitamin E through diet or pills can reduce the incidence of heart attack by 75%. The most common sources of dietary vitamin E are mayonnaise and margarine! "But aren't these foods notoriously high in fat?" You know darn well they are. The news media really ran with this one. So, what is the best course? Well, it's not bologna sandwiches with tons of mayo. Prevention is still the answer.

Iron and CVD

I'll bet you didn't know that too much iron in your body can cause heart disease. A recent five-year study in Finland of 1,931 men reported that high

Table 5-3	
MAJOR FOOD SOURCES OF ANTIOXIDANT VITAMINS	
Vitamin E	Green leafy vegetables, sweet potatoes, avocado, vegetable oils, margarine, olives, nuts, seeds, wheat germ
Beta-carotene	Carrots, pumpkin, sweet potatoes, spinach, collard greens, apricots, cantaloupe, mangos
Vitamin C	Citrus fruits, cantaloupe, strawberries, raw leafy vegetables, cabbage, tomatoes, green peppers

levels of iron stores are a strong risk factor for heart disease. The researchers felt that too much iron was possibly a stronger risk factor than high blood pressure, high cholesterol, or diabetes. It could partly explain why women are relatively immune to heart attacks prior to menopause. During the menstrual years, monthly blood loss tends to keep iron stores low, but after menopause, iron levels rise rapidly. The Finnish researchers suggested that women could possibly control this postmenopausal risk by donating blood about about three times per year. More definitive studies need to be done before a serious recommendation of blood donation can be made. Meanwhile, current opinion is that iron supplements are not recommended for menopausal women unless there is a proven and specific need.

Summing Up

The 900-pound gorilla called cardiovascular disease can also be controlled by a number of lifestyle changes including proper diet, exercise, cessation of cigarette smoking, moderation in alcohol consumption, stress control, and monitoring for high blood pressure, elevated cholesterol, and diabetes. These issues are covered in Section III.

There is no cure available for cardiovascular disease at this time. Our best bet is to prevent it, or at least to lower the risks by adopting a healthy-heart lifestyle . . . preferably *before* menopause. If you have not done so already though, don't get all guilty and wimp out on me. Even if you have been a weak-willed, spineless jellyfish, you can still make it all better. So press on, dear reader, the prevention details are in Section III. At this point, however, we will continue with another of the low profile but serious threats of menopause: osteoporosis.

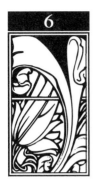

OSTEOPOROSIS
BONE BURGLARS AT WORK

Osteoporosis claims many lives and disables huge numbers of women because of bone loss and the resulting fractures. This chapter will teach you what osteoporosis is, who gets it, what happens to you, how to diagnose it, and how to prevent it.

Osteoporosis is the LOL (little old lady) maker. You've seen her everywhere, struggling along with her stooped back and her tentative gait to accomplish with great difficulty the things that formerly were routine and easy. At 80, she is three inches shorter than she was at 50, and she appears fragile, frail, and bent. Figure 6-1 illustrates the progressive changes in the spine that osteoporosis can cause over a 20-year period.

It does not have to happen to you because it is mostly preventable. Osteoporosis is the condition that results from loss of bone mass, a loss that actually starts in the mid-30s. Only minuscule, but detectable, amounts of bone are lost before menopause, but within six months of becoming menopausal, bone loss rapidly accelerates. The accelerated loss lasts for about five years, before leveling off to slower, but continuing, deterioration (Lindsay 1978).

A Little Bone Talk

Bone is living tissue, and like all living tissue, it is in a state of dynamic change. Bone tissue is being added and removed all the time. Normally there is a

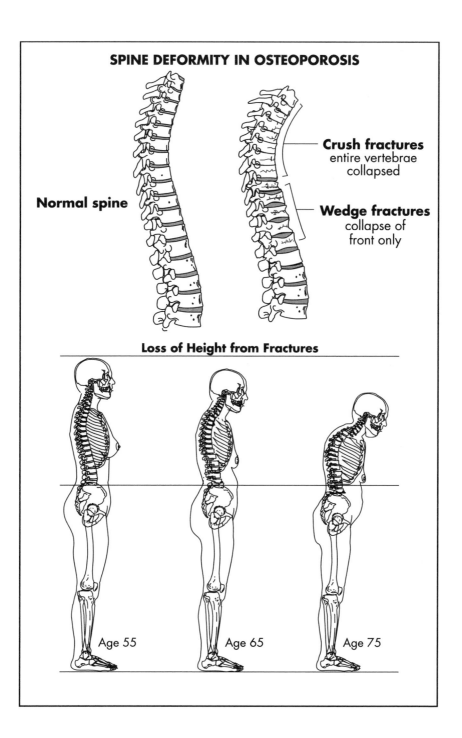

SPINE DEFORMITY IN OSTEOPOROSIS

Normal spine

Crush fractures
entire vertebrae
collapsed

Wedge fractures
collapse of
front only

Loss of Height from Fractures

Age 55

Age 65

Age 75

balance established that results in your having a sturdy skeleton. When female hormone is removed, the bone removers start getting ahead of the bone replacers. This results in bones that are brittle and easily broken. Bones get their strength from protein fibers, which are combined with calcium phosphate crystals. A net loss of both bone protein and calcium is what causes osteoporosis.

SOME STAGGERING NUMBERS

Twenty-five million Americans have osteoporosis and 80% of them are women. According to the National Osteoporosis Foundation (NOF), one in every two women over age 50 will suffer an osteoporotic fracture during her lifetime. One-third of all women over 65 will suffer one or more compression fractures of the vertebrae because of osteoporosis. This amounts to over 500,000 vertebral crush fractures annually. Refer to Figure 6-1 for the effects of compression vertebral fractures on posture and height as you age. Every year, over 250,000 women sustain hip fractures from osteoporosis. Of these women, 15%–20% die within three months from surgical complications and/or heart and lung problems associated with the resulting immobility. As many as half are dead within a year, and up to 50% of the survivors are permanently disabled (Speroff 1989). A postmenopausal woman's risk of hip fracture is as great as the risk of breast, uterine, and ovarian cancer *combined*.

Osteoporosis results in 1.3 million fractures annually from all skeletal sites. It is a major factor in the rapidly rising number of women who require nursing home care. Indeed, 75% of nursing home residents over age 65 are women. The cost for medical care is $10 billion, in addition to the appalling human toll. Unless prevention methods are more widely understood and utilized, osteoporotic fractures will be of epidemic proportions when the boomer generation matures into the postmenopausal years. Treatment of osteoporosis is now available; however, it is of limited value, so prevention is still the best game in town.

WHO'S AT RISK AND WHO ISN'T

The following are factors that increase the risk of osteoporosis:

✦ race. Caucasians and Asians suffer more often from osteoporosis than do blacks. Black women produce increased levels of calcitonin, a hormone secreted in your thyroid that stimulates bone formation
✦ fair skin and blond hair
✦ thin women with petite frames. In women with more body fat, a process called *aromatization* produces some estrogen from body fat, independent of the ovaries. This is not an obesity recommenda-

tion, because the risk of heart disease and high blood pressure in obesity outweigh the benefit of a peripheral estrogen source from body fat. But the "fashion-model" body style puts you at greater risk of bone loss

✦ premature menopause, especially under age 40, either spontaneous or surgical. The risk factor is simply that there are many more years to live without the protection of estrogen

✦ family history of osteoporosis, one of the most important risk factors

✦ tobacco use of one half pack or more per day and/or alcohol consumption of 5 ounces or more per day (maybe even less)

✦ sedentary lifestyle. Healthy bones require weight-bearing activity

✦ hyperthyroidism or hyperparathyroidism, meaning overactivity by the thyroid or parathyroid gland

✦ diet low in calcium, especially as a child or young adult

✦ prior dieting as an adult with a high protein, low carbohydrate regimen

✦ late menarche. Onset of menstrual periods after age 16 means several teen years with inadequate estrogen

✦ no full-term pregnancies, i.e., never had a prolonged estrogen surge

✦ long-term corticosteroid (cortisone) use, which can result in 30% bone loss within six months

✦ prolonged depression. This increases the risk for osteoporosis because of increased levels of the stress hormone cortisol. Bone density is 10%–15% lower in depressed women, according to Dr. Philip Gold, a neuroendocrinologist at the National Institute of Mental Health

✦ immune system abnormalities. People with autoimmune diseases such as rheumatoid arthritis have more osteoporosis. Dr. Louis V. Avioli at Washington University School of Medicine in St. Louis says that certain bone marrow substances called *cytokines* can get out of control and increase bone breakdown

Diminished risk of osteoporosis is seen in these situations:

✦ muscular or overweight women
✦ several term pregnancies
✦ oral contraceptive pill users
✦ estrogen use at menopause

Osteoporosis is a slow, silent process which does not result in symptoms until well established. By the time it is well established, it is only partially reversible. The peak bone density is generally reached by the late 20s. Up to that time, a positive balance has been in effect, meaning more replacement than removal of bone protein and calcium. The peak bone density for specifically the vertebrae and most other bones is reached in the late 20s (Avioli 1984). For the radius (forearm bone), loss does not start to become measurable until about one year after menopause (Johnston 1985).

In industrialized societies over the past three decades, the actual density of bone has been declining in women. In Oslo, Norway, for example, there were five times more fractures in 1982 than in 1950; researchers felt that it was because of the marked cutback in consumption of dairy products (Felch 1985). This emphasizes the importance of dietary calcium and protein. But do not be misled: *estrogen* is the engine that gets utilization of the calcium and protein accomplished. Even with adequate calcium and protein intake the fracture rate is not lowered without estrogen in the equation. There are two widely held misconceptions about osteoporosis: first that it is easy to prevent, and second that once you are five or 10 years beyond menopause, there is no value in starting estrogen. Neither is true. More on these two points later.

Prevention, the Best Game in Town

Well, all of the above certainly establishes the bone burglar as one dangerous dude, but not to worry. Don't forget, I said this is a largely preventable situation. Osteoporosis is not a disease process. You can't "catch it." You can't as yet completely cure it either, but there is plenty you can do to reduce your risk.

REDUCING YOUR RISK

One of the major opportunities to avoid the risk of postmenopausal osteoporosis occurs between the ages of 11 to 24. This window is largely unknown or ignored. During this time, bones are growing and bone mass is accumulating to reach its peak in the late 20s. To reach their peak bone mass, adolescents and young adult women must have a calcium intake of 1,200–1,500 mg per day. A glass of milk or serving of yogurt has about 300 mg of calcium. That would be a start. They also need 400 IU of vitamin D daily (100 IU per glass of milk), adequate exercise, and adequate estrogen.

Most teenage and young adult women do indeed have plenty of estrogen. I'm sure you remember your "rampaging hormone" era. If not, consult your mother. She'll remember it for sure. Estrogen may be too low in some young women from a delayed onset of menstrual periods or a prolonged absence of periods for any reason. If any or all of these four necessary "ingredients" (calcium, Vitamin D, exercise, estrogen) is absent for a long time during these years, the peak bone mass may never be reached (Theistz 1992). This is the person who will be at greater risk for osteoporosis later in life. So, tell your daughters about this, and, at the grave risk of appearing meddlesome, tell your granddaughters too.

At age 50, life expectancy is about another 32 years, and the risk of osteoporotic fracture comes late in those years. For hip and wrist fractures, the lifetime risk is one in six. For vertebrae it is one in four. When you are 50 years old, it may seem a bit far-fetched to be worrying about an event that could be three decades in the future, but other changes in the quality of your life will evolve (loss of height, pain, frailness) if you do nothing to avoid them. Prevention must start now.

PREVENTION WITH ESTROGEN

I guess you knew that hormone replacement was going to get in here somewhere. Actually, there is much more than HRT that helps your prevention program, but HRT is of primary importance (Prince 1991). With it, a 50%–60% decrease in wrist and hip fractures can be expected (Kiel 1987). If calcium is added, an 80% reduction in compression fractures of vertebrae results.

Estrogen not only helps you absorb calcium better, it also has a direct effect on bone formation itself. The bone removers are called *osteoclasts*. Bone replacers are called *osteoblasts*, and it is known that osteoblasts have estrogen receptors. This means that when estrogen occupies the receptor sites, it stimulates osteoblasts to form bone, hence the reason that estrogen is so important to bone integrity. The exact mechanism of osteoblast stimulation is still unknown, but by golly, it works, and that is known.

WHAT ABOUT PROGESTIN?

Well, all that happy talk about estrogen is just fine, you're thinking; but what about progestin? In Chapter 5 it was stated that progestin is an anti-estrogen. Won't it prevent estrogen from preventing osteoporosis? Turns out that it won't interfere. Dr. J. A. Cauley and others published a study in 1995 of 9,704 women over age 65 showing no difference in fracture rate between those who used unopposed estrogen and those who used combined estrogen-progestin. This strongly suggests that progestin has no adverse effect. As a matter of fact, progestin, even if given alone, will reduce bone removal. And get *this*: When progestin is added to estrogen, it actually *increases* bone formation slightly (Abdella 1985, Selby 1985, Christianson 1985). How about *that*, folks?

Estrogen and progesterone protection against osteoporosis lasts as long as the hormones are in your body. When withdrawn by menopause or by quitting HRT, accelerated bone loss begins. It will last about five years, before leveling off to continuing but slower loss. Former HRT users have almost the same rate of fractures as women who *never* took HRT. Therefore the practice of using HRT for only the first 10 years after menopause is a waste of resources and definitely to be discouraged. So, for the maximum protection against fractures, HRT needs to be started soon after hormone production declines and should be taken for the long term. Even if not started until after age 75, there is improved bone formation for about one to three years. Newer drugs (bisphosphonates) can improve this picture. They are discussed below. Though complete retrieval of lost bone does not happen in the elderly woman, her protection against fractures is improved by about one-third, and it will persist if she continues HRT. For women on lifelong HRT, fracture risk is cut by two-thirds!

MALE HORMONE PLUS ESTROGEN

A 1996 study by Dr. L. G. Raisz published in the *Journal of Clinical Endocrinology* demonstrated that combining estrogen and testosterone caused an increase in bone formation, as compared to estrogen's ability only to prevent bone loss. This is encouraging, but the study was rather small and left unanswered the question as to whether long-term use of male hormone would decrease the good guy HDL as it does in men. This would increase the risk of cardiovascular disease. Preliminary indications are that it will not when used in small doses. The answer? More study is needed.

MORE PREVENTION HELP: CALCIUM

In real estate it's location, location, location. For osteoporosis it's prevention, prevention, prevention, because a skeleton is a terrible thing to waste.

Calcium needs more explanation. From menopause onward, women taking estrogen need about 1,000 mg of calcium each day. Nonusers need 1,500 mg per day. See Table 6-1 for daily calcium needs throughout the life cycle. The average daily intake of calcium from diet is only 500 mg; so a supplement of 500 mg is needed. For women who are menopausal and not on HRT, a supplement of 1,000 mg is needed since calcium absorption from your intestine is significantly diminished after menopause, especially after age 60. Higher doses, especially beyond 2,000 mg, have little impact on bone mass in the absence of estrogen-progestin. Higher doses of calcium also cause annoying problems like constipation and gas.

Other important information to know about calcium is that it is utilized by your brain, your muscles, your heart, the blood clotting mechanism, and in many other vital body functions on an ongoing daily basis. Calcium is so vital to normal bodily functioning that an elaborate hormone system is constantly regulating its level in your blood. This system involves parathyroid hormone, calcitonin hormone from the thyroid, vitamin D, reproductive hormones (estrogen, progesterone, androgen), and adrenal gland hormones (glucocor-

Table 6-1

DAILY CALCIUM REQUIREMENTS FOR NORMAL BONE MASS

Age group	Needed daily
11–25 years	1,200–1,500 mg
25–50	1,000 mg
Pregnant or breastfeeding	1,200–1,500 mg
Over 50	
Taking estrogen	1,000 mg
No estrogen	1,500 mg
Over 65	1,500 mg

ticoids). If your daily calcium intake is inadequate, your body gets the needed amount from its storage depot—your bones. Over time, if a deficit in calcium intake persists, it results in a less sturdy skeleton. The deficit increases with aging because calcium absorption becomes less efficient. Since the average American woman's food preferences do not supply enough calcium, the majority of you will need a calcium supplement (Nachtigall 1995).

Dietary calcium and calcium supplements require some thought and coordination, if you are to get the most benefit. Look over the list of foods in Table 6-2 for their calcium content. Notice that some of the foods that are high in calcium are also high in calories or in fat content. Examples are sardines, nuts, or ice cream. So you need to pick and choose a bit. The following list of important suggestions for calcium intake will help clarify calcium utilization for you.

✦ You can only absorb about 600 mg of calcium at a time. It is best to take it in divided doses throughout the day if your daily need is more than that amount. Take your calcium supplement with meals, because you have a better hydrochloric acid content in your stomach at that time. This prevents stomach irritation from the calcium. Do not take more calcium than your daily need, because the excess will only be excreted by your kidneys. An excess will interfere with your body's absorption of iron and zinc, and it can also cause constipation and gas.

✦ Drink plenty of water every day. It helps in the absorption of calcium.

✦ Aluminum-containing antacids (alhydroxides) take calcium out of your body. Do not use them on a regular basis or as a calcium supplement. Examples are Gelusil, Amphogel, Maalox Plus Tablets, Mylanta Liquid, and Tempo. Products *without* aluminum include Tums, Riopan, Mylanta Gelcaps, Mylanta Double Strength, Maalox Antacid Caplets, Titralac, Rolaids, and Alkamints.

Table 6-2

CALCIUM CONTENT IN VARIOUS FOODS

Food		Serving	Calcium	Calories	Fat grams
Milk					
	Whole	1 cup	288 mg	150	8.1
	Skim	1 cup	296 mg	89	4.7
Cheese					
	Cheddar	1 oz.	204 mg	112	9.1
	Swiss	1 oz.	260 mg	95	7.1
	Cottage, low fat, 2%	4 oz.	78 mg	100	2.2
Yogurt					
	Whole milk	1 cup	274 mg	141	7.7
	Plain, low fat	1 cup	414 mg	143	3.4
Ice cream, 10% fat					
	Hard (vanilla)	1 cup	176 mg	270	14.1
	Soft (vanilla)	1 cup	236 mg	375	25.6
Ice milk					
	Hard, 4% fat (vanilla)	1 cup	176 mg	185	4.6
	Soft, 3% fat (vanilla)	1 cup	274 mg	225	8.6
Tofu					
	Firm curd	4 oz.	6–100 mg	150	8
	Medium curd	4 oz.	4–90 mg	90	6
Vegetables					
	Spinach, fresh, cooked, drained	1 cup	150 mg	40	0
	Broccoli, fresh, cooked, drained	1 cup	136 mg	40	0
	Lima beans, fresh, cooked	½ cup	81 mg	120	0
	Collards, fresh, cooked, drained	1 cup	357 mg	65	0
	Turnip greens, fresh, cooked	1 cup	252 mg	30	0
Seafood					
	Shrimp, canned, drained	3½ oz.	115 mg	100	0.8
	Salmon, canned, with bones	3½ oz.	183 mg	210	14
	Oysters, raw, 18 medium size	3½ oz.	258 mg	160	2.0
	Sardines, canned, with bones	3½ oz.	425 mg	311	24.4
Nuts & Seeds					
	Almonds, shelled, about 12 nuts	1 oz.	45 mg	170	15
	Sunflower seeds, hulled	1 oz.	35 mg	159	14

Adapted from National Osteoporosis Foundation

✦ Regular use of laxatives can interfere with calcium absorption because laxatives speed up the passage time of food through your body. Same is true for bulk forming stool softeners if they are taken at the same time as calcium supplements. A very high fiber diet has the same effect. You need the fiber though, so don't take your calcium supplement with a high-fiber meal.

✦ Green leafy vegetables (turnip greens, spinach, Swiss chard) block calcium absorption. Although these vegetables are loaded with calcium, they contain oxalic acid which inhibits calcium absorption, as well as of other nutrients. They may appear to be an attractive source of calcium, but you will fail to get the maximum calcium benefit when you consume them. They may also block the benefit of other calcium sources, when ingested at the same time.

✦ Calcium interferes with iron absorption, so don't take these supplements together.

✦ Avoid calcium-enriched "juice drinks," because they usually only contain about 10% juice. Instead use real juice that is fortified with calcium—usually about 300 mg of calcium citrate.

✦ A high fat diet decreases calcium absorption, and so does a large intake of zinc or megadoses of vitamin A.

After studying Table 6-2 and the preceding list of do's and don'ts regarding calcium use, it becomes obvious that it is not really possible to get your daily requirement of 1,500 mg without a calcium supplement. (There's just too much milk to drink, or too many oysters to eat.) On the other hand, if your daily dietary calcium intake is indeed adequate, you probably don't need a supplement until your 60s when your ability to absorb calcium begins to decline.

SELECTING A CALCIUM SUPPLEMENT

All of the supplements contain calcium, of course, but it is important to know the *bioavailability* of the calcium. You can find this on the label of the bottle, where it discloses the amount of *elemental calcium* per tablet. This is the amount available for absorption into your body.

Calcium carbonate is generally the best choice since it has the highest amount of elemental calcium; it is usually cheaper than other forms too. It can cause constipation and gas, so take it with whichever of your meals are low in fiber. Oyster shell calcium has been a popular supplement for calcium carbonate because it is organic, but it is more expensive and not any more useful than others. There are many antacids that utilize calcium carbonate, but it is best to avoid the ones that contain aluminum, which promotes calcium loss. Just shop the shelves for the cheapest one that has the most bioavailable calcium.

Examples to look for are Caltrate, Os-Cal, Tums-Ex, Calcium Rich Rolaids, oyster shell.

Calcium citrate works quite well because it is more readily broken down in the stomach and therefore more completely absorbed. It has only about half as much bioavailability as calcium carbonate, so more tablets must be taken and this makes it more expensive. If you are over 65, this may be the best form to take because you have less stomach acid. Citracal is a good brand to look for.

Calcium phosphate marketed as Posture has about the same bioavailability and absorption characteristics as calcium carbonate. The main difference is that it is more expensive.

Calcium gluconate and *calcium lactate* both have low levels of bioavailability, requiring many more tablets to be taken and increasing the cost up to 10 times.

Some brands do not readily dissolve in your stomach, which dramatically reduces their usefulness. A good test for this is to immerse a tablet in vinegar; it should dissolve to powder in half an hour. If not, you got a bad one. Be sure to tell your pharmacist about it.

Magnesium and calcium have similar functions in your body in muscle contraction and nerve-impulse transmission. They are commonly combined in supplements. An excess of one can cause inhibition of the other, so your *magnesium intake should never be more than half of calcium*. If your daily calcium supplement is 1,000 mg, your magnesium should not be more than 500 mg. Food sources are seafood, nuts, fresh green leafy vegetables, cereal grains, figs, corn, apples, and soybeans.

Phosphorus is a major component of bone. Too much of it leads to bone loss by stimulating the parathyroid gland hormone to remove calcium from bone. Rotten trick, but that's the parathyroid's job. Major dietary sources of phosphorus are cola drinks, red meats, and processed foods which contain phosphorus additives, so moderation in phosphorous intake is essential.

Vitamin D is known to increase the absorption of calcium from the intestinal tract and is therefore recommended. That is good news for getting calcium aboard, but it is also known that without estrogen the fracture rate is not reduced in spite of adequate vitamin D and calcium (Riggs 1982). If the increased absorption does not lead to increased utilization of calcium in bones, high levels of calcium accumulate in the blood stream and can lead to kidney stones. The kidney stone risk is not as great as had formerly been thought, and some recent research suggests calcium citrate in adequate amounts may actually help prevent them. Until more is known, *too much vitamin D is to be avoided*. The recommended daily intake is 400 IU/day, especially if you live where there are cloudy winters and get less vitamin D from sunlight. Ten to fifteen minutes of sunshine exposure daily will produce adequate vitamin D for most. Elderly women who do not get out much usually need 800 IU/day.

Some New Products for Prevention and Treatment

Calcitonin is a hormone produced by your thyroid gland; it prevents bone loss if you have an adequate calcium intake. After menopause, however, the amount of natural calcitonin produced is not sufficient to protect you from osteoporosis. Scientists have produced a synthetic form of calcitonin, based on the type that salmon make, that is 15 times more potent than the human hormone. It has been shown to gradually increase bone mass by as much as 5%–20%. It also decreases the pain of vertebral fractures in women who have severe osteoporosis. A nasal spray has been available in 72 countries for several years, and the FDA finally approved it for use in the United States in late 1995. The spray is marketed by Sandoz Pharmaceuticals Corporation under the name Miacalcin. Clinical studies indicated that daily calcitonin-salmon nasal spray significantly increases spinal bone density, but has minimal bone-building effect on the hip and forearms, which are common sites for fractures. There are side effects such as nasal irritation, dryness, itching, and bleeding. The injectable form also has side effects including nausea, vomiting, skin rash, abdominal pain, diarrhea, and facial flushing. Calcitonin is a good addition to our armory in the battle against the bone burglars, but it doesn't work as well as prevention.

Bisphophonates are a type of drug you may not have heard about. These drugs are absorbed into the bone where they remain permanently and decrease your osteoclasts' ability to remove bone tissue. This gives your osteoblasts a tilted playing field and a more unimpeded chance to build bone. The first generation of this drug, called *etidronate* and marketed as Didronel, has been shown to increase bone mass, especially in the spine, by 5% in two years. Other bones, like wrists and hips, were less improved. Didronel is taken in a 400 mg dose for two weeks every three months, and with few side effects. If taken with estrogen, there is an additive effect on your formation of new bone mass.

A new second generation of bisphosphonates, *alendronate* and *pamidronate*, are showing promise as a nonhormonal method for not only preventing but also *treating* osteoporosis. Alendronate was marketed in late 1995 under the name Fosamax. Like Didronel, it works by preventing bone removal and allowing bone formation to proceed unimpeded. Studies of four to six years duration thus far have shown that a 10 mg daily dose resulted in a 6%–10% increase in bone density within three years, and increased bone *strength* as well! The vertebral fracture rates were reduced by nearly 50%. In contrast to Didronel, Fosamax has its effect on *all* bones. A downside is that Fosamax is poorly absorbed from the intestine unless taken with a full eight-ounce glass of water, after eight hours of fasting. You must avoid *anything* else in your stomach for at least a half hour and ideally two hours after taking it. Well then why not take it at bedtime? you might thoughtfully inquire. Because you probably will not have been fasting for as much as eight hours, and because you absolutely must not lie down while Fosamax is in your stomach. It can cause ferocious irritation of your esophagus (heartburn) if you get yourself horizontal. To be effective, it must be used continuously and long term. It probably can be used with estrogen, but no long-term studies have as yet shown this. Since Fosamax has no protective effect on CVD, estrogen will likely be prescribed for you if you wish to take it. As for pamidronate, it has been shown to increase bone density and decrease fractures associated with osteoporosis (Speroff 1997). It must be given by intravenous solution about once monthly.

Sodium fluoride is being investigated as a treatment for osteoporosis by Dr. Charles Yak at Texas Southwestern Medical Center. It is in a new slow-release combination with calcium citrate. Fluorides in high doses were used in the 1980s to treat osteoporosis, but it actually resulted in a higher fracture rate. There was good bone density but lousy bone strength. This new method may increase bone mass by more than 4% over four years, but more research is needed because the difference between toxicity and effectiveness is rather narrow.

Some Old but Important Points on Prevention

Cessation of cigarette smoking is standard advice now because it is well established that smoking causes an earlier menopause and an increased risk of osteoporosis—among many other health risks. Studies have now shown that smoking inhibits the ovarian follicle cells from producing adequate female hormone, which leads to an earlier menopause. In addition, smoking causes changes in the estrogen that is produced, so that it cannot be properly utilized by your body. The lower level of useful estrogen even before menopause results in reduced bone density. When menopause does come to smokers, HRT in the usual dosage is not capable of fully counteracting this smoking effect. For postmenopausal smokers, estrogen blood levels should be checked because higher doses of HRT may be needed to maintain the desired 60–100 pg/ml level (Hopper 1994).

Exercise is a real must in preventing and/or managing osteoporosis. Weight-bearing movement increases bone mass, no question about it. Being a couch potato reduces bone mass. Due to an absence of weight-bearing exercise, astronauts start suffering bone loss when they are out in space, weightless. The bone reducers (osteoclasts) get right to work on those space walkers, ripping out bone and sending the calcium levels in their urine sky high . . . or into orbit, if you prefer.

There are three forms of exercise: too much, too little, and just enough. Just enough can be as little as 30 minutes of brisk walking three times per week, although four to five times is better. The essential value of exercise is not only that it improves bone mass and prevents fractures, but also that it strengthens muscle. This improves balance and helps prevent falls, a potential problem if you already have osteoporosis.

The risk of excessive exercise for women who are not yet menopausal is that the hypothalamus may become suppressed and interrupt the menstrual cycle. This causes low ovarian hormone production and osteoporosis. As mentioned earlier in this book, it takes very heavy exercise to do this, such as what a world-class runner would do. For women who already have osteoporosis, too much exercise can cause fractures. Jogging is too damaging to joint surfaces, but walking, which is low impact, is fine. Exercising in water is particularly helpful for strengthening muscles without undue stress on weakened or previously fractured bones; however, it won't help prevent osteoporosis because you experience diminished weight bearing in water. The trick is to find a balance between beneficial levels of exercise that will stimulate new bone formation and exercise levels that risk fractures. The benefit of exercise on the compressed bones which result from vertebral osteoporosis is less than that for long bones, so it is especially important for osteoporotic women to be on hormone replacement and calcium supplementation (Speroff 1989). More on exercise in Chapter 14.

Alcoholics have long been known to be at risk for osteoporosis. The questions have always been why is that so and how much is too much? The why has yet to be answered, but suspicion centers around alcohol preventing absorption of calcium and vitamin D. Poor nutrition and a decrease in your liver's ability to activate vitamin D are also suspected. As for how much, as few as three drinks per day on a regular basis may result in low bone mass, so the current wisdom is to limit alcohol consumption to two drinks per day or less. Some say that two to six drinks per week puts you at risk for a hip fracture. You are definitely at risk of fracture if your consumption is sufficient to lose your balance and fall. If *you* get smashed, your bones can too.

Caffeine is on the hit list too. In the Nurse's Health Study, postmenopausal women who had more than four cups of coffee per day were shown to have a tripling of their risk for hip fracture. Another study showed that women who drank two cups per day had normal bone density if they also had a glass of milk each day. So if you need a morning jolt of coffee, keep calcium in mind.

Certain medications in long-term or excessive use inhibit calcium absorption and/or utilization. These include high doses of anticonvulsants, lithium, tetracycline, cortisone and similar steroids, certain diuretics like Lasix, fiber preparations such as Metamucil, antacids containing aluminum, and high doses of thyroid hormone.

New breakthroughs in nonhormonal drug therapy to prevent osteoporosis are on the horizon: for example, Smith Kline Beecham has discovered a gene on osteoclasts that promotes bone removal. The search is now under way for a method to block this genetic effect.

How Do I Know If I've Got It?

Diagnosing osteoporosis should be easy, right? Just get your bones x-rayed. But alas, it is not that simple. What needs to be known is how *dense* your bones are. Standard X rays do not indicate any abnormalities in density until you have already lost about 30%–40%. By then, it is already too late for a complete retrieval of lost bone. A more sensitive test of density can be done with *dual energy X-ray absorptiometry* (DEXA). This is a scanner that can measure as little as a 1% loss of density.

But what about the excess radiation we are told to avoid? The average adult American receives 3,000 units of natural radiation (measured in a unit called uSV) from the atmosphere each year. A DEXA scan will add one uSV to that total. A computed tomography (CT) scan also works, but requires more radiation than with DEXA and will not measure the femur (thigh bone). DEXA seems to be the procedure of choice because it evaluates all three sites of interest: wrist, hip, and spine. Its cost is about $175–$200 and declining.

Ultrasound (US) may have a role to play in diagnosis, since US measurements of bone density in the heel bone and knee cap are known to correlate fairly well with the true state of osteoporosis by DEXA methods. And, ultrasound is much less expensive.

Measuring bone mass on a routine basis is generally not indicated in every postmenopausal woman, but this is a controversial topic. It is not cost-effective from the perspective of the medical economists. In addition, most post-menopausal women who have low risk factors and are on HRT to begin with would not likely have their treatment plan changed by the DEXA result. On the other hand, a younger perimenopausal woman who is at known risk for osteoporosis (family history of osteoporosis, very thin, smoker, poor diet, no exercise) can benefit from the results of a DEXA by adopting an aggressive prevention program should her bone density be below normal. Under these circumstances the cost effectiveness of DEXA becomes obvious; a woman is able to prevent the huge future expense of fracture treatment, rehabilitation, and perhaps long-term nursing home care.

Speroff recommends bone density measurement in three specific situations:

1. When a woman needs the information in order to make an informed decision about HRT. For example, how much osteoporosis, if any, do

I now have? For women who have very sturdy skeletons, it may not be necessary to start HRT immediately at menopause.

2. To measure the effectiveness of treatment in special situations, such as with smokers, long-term thyroid hormone use, and long-term corticosteroid use. All of these factors cause rapid bone loss.

3. To measure bone loss in women whose HRT use and attention to prevention details have been spotty. If bone density loss has continued, showing her this may motivate her to get with the program (Speroff 1995).

Summing Up

The bottom line for dealing with osteoporosis is that while calcium supplements, weight-bearing exercise, quitting smoking, and other modalities are all helpful in maintaining bone density, you really need hormone replacement therapy to lower the fracture rate. Should all menopausal women use hormone replacement therapy? Not if you have normal bone density, you exercise regularly, you don't smoke, you maintain good nutrition, and there are no other risk factors for you. If you elect not to use HRT, your bone density should be monitored closely about once a year in the first five years after menopause.

At this point in time, prevention is the best game in town, and being aggressive is the only way to play it. Why? Because prevention is successful if started well before the onset of menopause, and also because once significant bone loss has occurred, complete retrieval can never be accomplished. If you snooze, you lose. Actually, prevention ideally should start in the teens, but if you are reading this book, it's a pretty safe bet that you are not a teenager. Am I right? That said about prevention, I must also reiterate that new nonhormonal products have recently been introduced (second generation bisphosphonates) not only to prevent osteoporosis, but also to treat it. Your doctor should be able to discuss those options with you as you design your osteoporosis prevention plan.

Osteoporosis affects a very large number of women who are living many postmenopausal years. It constitutes a huge public health problem. Successful prevention can have a major impact on the health care system, as well as on you personally in terms of medical expense, quality of life, and avoidance of premature death.

For more information about osteoporosis contact the

National Osteoporosis Foundation
2100 M Street NW
Washington, D.C. 20037
(202) 223-3336

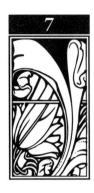

CANCER AND HORMONES
WHAT'S KNOWN AND WHAT ISN'T

In the past two decades, considerable fear has been generated regarding the relationship between hormone replacement and cancer. Some of it is justified and some not. Published articles have cited studies that were poorly done, where the data collected were misinterpreted by the authors and the conclusions, sensationalized by medically unsophisticated print and broadcast media. The result, of course, has been that the public has become frightened, and many people have declined treatment that could have helped them. This chapter is about two hot button issues: the relationship between breast cancer and hormone use and the relationship between uterine cancer and hormone use.

The two most common reasons for menopausal women to decline HRT, or to discontinue it, are

1. irregular uterine bleeding (or even regular bleeding)
2. fear of cancer

Both are valid reasons. Bleeding can be controlled with known and proven methods; but fear of cancer can only be relieved by accurate knowledge of the risks, plus prevention and cure. This chapter will summarize for you most of the current published knowledge about the association of hormone therapy with uterine and breast cancer. First, some background information about cancer cells and what causes them.

What Is Cancer and Why Do We Get It?

Cancer is an abnormality in individual cells. Each cancer cell has acquired the abnormality and will convey it to its daughter cells. Normal cells all have genes that control how the cell functions, when it reproduces itself, and when it dies. Over time, the genes controlling the cell may become altered by aging, as well as by toxic agents we consume or to which we become exposed. This alteration is called *mutation*. After a mutation has occurred, the altered gene is copied in all subsequent cell reproduction. If the mutation has produced a cancer-causing gene, called an *oncogene*, then succeeding generations of that cell all have the potential to become cancer cells. Some people are born with oncogenes already in place, which stay dormant until stimulated into activity by things like aging and bodily exposures to environmental irritants. Once the oncogene is activated, the cell no longer behaves in a normal fashion. It becomes a rogue cell with uncontrolled growth and invades the territory of normal neighboring tissues and organs. Cancer cells, with their changed genetic prescription, cannot perform the same functions as normal cells, so the body suffers as these functions are lost. Without effective treatment to halt the unchecked growth of cancer cells, death is the outcome.

There may be some future help in this regard. In the past two years, cancer biologists have identified a protein called *telomerase*. It is a chemical produced by cancer cells that confers immortality to the cancer cell. With telomerase, cancer cells can divide over and over without succumbing to aging and death as normal cells behave. Telomerase can be detected in about 85% of cancers. In breast and lung cancer, it can be detected even before the tumor has started to spread. The problem so far is that telomerase can only be detected from the tissue cells themselves, so a biopsy is needed. A blood test will not work; therefore, telomerase testing would not be useful as a mass screening tool. About a dozen pharmaceutical companies are working on drugs to shut down telomerase, which of course would starve the cancer cells of a chemical they need to survive. This is certainly one of the most exciting breakthroughs in cancer biology in the past decade.

WHY DON'T WE KNOW MORE?

I will try to set the record straight for you, but you will see that many unknowns remain, partially because studies under way have yet to be completed. In my research for this book, I came across many comments by professional writers who savaged the medical establishment for not knowing more about menopause, hormone replacement, or female cancer. Of course, more needs to be known, and it is reassuring that much more *will* be known. But that the needed information is not yet available is attributable to several factors:

✦ Time is not the least of them. It takes lots of time to get valid results that are statistically significant. For example, to the consternation of many observers, a number of questions are pending regarding what effect birth control pills, taken over the past three and a half decades, will have on postmenopausal women. The pill became available in the early 1960s, and the early pill users are just now becoming post-menopausal in large numbers. Some answers are only now becoming available. So the question is, Should the pill have been withheld from the public for the past 35 years pending completion of the research? Or is it prudent or justifiable to use short-term research to make predictions on safety and efficacy? The late Yul Brenner said it in his movie *The King and I*: "Is a puzzlement."

✦ Research priorities have been set by urgency. The public, and there-fore the scientific community, has been more concerned with the problems of old age (CVD, cancer, arthritis) and of early age (prema-turity, birth defects, childhood diseases) than with the problems of middle age. Most people in the middle years are healthy. The prob-lems that do exist for these women and men have not been regarded by the public as more urgent than those of the other age groups.

✦ Money is a major factor. Research is expensive, and money has not been unlimited. This equation results in strategic decisions having to be made as to where to spend the funds. Sixty years ago the major thrust was to control infections which killed millions with impunity. Antibiotic and vaccine research got the lion's share. Twenty-five years ago the government decided that infection was well under control, and cancer became the money favorite. More recently, AIDS is being increasingly perceived as the major threat. Menopausal problems and women's health issues never made the headlines or the evening news. So menopause remained in the closet, and its discussion continued to be one of our cultural taboos. This book will not make menopause a headline either, but hopefully it will change its status in the minds of some, so that research and open communication about it may grow.

Uterine Cancer

Endometrial (uterine lining) cancer is the most common external or internal genital cancer in women over age 45. In the 1990s, approximately 33,000 new cases are being diagnosed each year with almost 6,000 deaths, making it the fourth most frequent female cancer of any type. Lung, breast, and colorectal (colon or rectum) cancer are the first three. In the '90s, the frequency of endometrial cancer has stabilized and may be decreasing.

This disease was not considered a serious risk for women on HRT until 1975, when two medical studies reported that estrogen increased the incidence of endometrial cancer. The reports triggered a decade or more of intense study, furious debate, and egregious arguments in the medical literature. Ultimately, the preponderance of evidence showed that the cancer increase was true. Estrogen was the culprit. It got nailed to the wall. But guess what else the research showed: If progestin is combined with estrogen, the increased risk is reversed.

THE PROGESTIN STORY AND ENDOMETRIAL CANCER

Present numbers on endometrial cancer indicate that of postmenopausal women who are not on HRT, about 1–2 women per 1,000 run the risk of getting this cancer each year. If estrogen is used alone (unopposed by progestin), the risk is 5–8 times higher, depending on the dose and duration of use (Speroff 1989). If progestin is added, the risk of cancer is reduced to the same as in women who use no hormones at all. A study by Gambrell in 1983 actually found that adding progestin reduced the risk of cancer to *less* than that in women who used no hormones at all. It was exciting news, but it was not confirmed by other researchers—a condition necessary to scientific acceptance.

The reason progestin helps is this: Estrogen causes growth of the endometrium in postmenopausal women, and progestin inhibits it. Progestin inhibits by reducing the number of available estrogen receptors on the endometrial cells and by inducing enzymes in the cell to change estrogen from estradiol (the most potent form of estrogen) to estrone (the least potent). The degree of estrogen stimulation of endometrial cells is thus greatly diminished, and that is the protective mechanism.

Women commonly ask, "Why not just do a hysterectomy after menopause, so I don't have to worry about cancer and I don't need to take progestin?" A good question. The answers are: 1) the operation is a major one with its own inherent risks (see Chapter 15) and major expense; 2) progestin use is effective, well tolerated by most, and not costly.

WHAT ARE MY RISKS?

Most of the risks for this cancer are associated with any situation that exposes your endometrial lining to prolonged estrogen stimulation without the protective influence of progesterone.

✦ Hormone replacement with estrogen only has already been mentioned. Recently, there has been some interest in using unopposed estrogen with the addition of two weeks of progestin every three months. This seems to be adequately protective of the endometrium, but long-term studies are not yet available.

✦ Anovulation, or absence of ovulation, puts you at risk because most of the progesterone you make occurs after ovulation. Failure to ovulate exposes you to unopposed estrogen. Several situations may create this risk:

1. prolonged infertility from anovulation
2. prolonged perimenopausal transition without ovulation
3. polycystic ovary syndrome results in abnormal estrogens, increased male hormone production, and anovulation or very irregular ovulation
4. teenage anovulation is a common early trait after periods begin and before normal ovulatory cycles start. It does not result from any particular abnormality, but if it lasts for months or years, these young girls will have increased lifetime risk for later endometrial cancer

✦ Obesity results in excess estrogen stimulation because of a process called *aromatization*, which creates estrone, a weak estrogen, from fat cells. Unlike the cyclic estrogen production by your ovaries, this is a constant source. The longer you are overweight, the greater your risk.

✦ Diabetes is an independent risk factor for endometrial cancer. Compounding the problem is the fact that many diabetics are overweight, which adds excess estrone production to the risk. Many diabetics also have high blood pressure, and this adds to the risk as well. A triple whammy.

✦ Tamoxifen is a drug used for the prevention of breast cancer recurrence. It does a good job, but it bears a close molecular resemblance to estrogen and can occupy estrogen receptor sites on endometrial cells. In that situation, it causes overgrowth of endometrial cells, called hyperplasia, which can lead to cancer. If you are on this drug, you need periodic ultrasound scanning of your endometrium to screen for any thickening.

SCREENING AND DIAGNOSIS

Ultrasound screening annually is a good idea if you have any of the risk factors listed above. This is done with a specially designed vaginal probe, which painlessly and accurately measures the thickness of your endometrial lining. A thickness measurement of 5mm or more suggests the possibility of hyperplasia, and tissue sampling will need to be done. If it is 4mm or less, you saved yourself an endometrial biopsy.

Tissue sampling for microscopic analysis is necessary for diagnosis. Abnormal bleeding or ultrasound findings are the triggers for suggesting this evaluation. There are basically three methods to obtain a tissue sample:

✦ *Dilation and Curettage* (D&C) was the time-honored method until the past decade or so. The technique involves dilation of the cervical canal and introduction of instruments to scrape tissue from the inside of your uterus. Since it is a blind procedure, meaning the doctor can't actually see the tissue to be removed, a D&C has some built-in inaccuracies. The operation is like trying to remove the inside of a pear by going through its neck. A D&C can miss polyps, fibroids, and even cancers. A diagnostic D&C is most commonly done in an operating room with the patient asleep. It is possible to do as an office procedure with local anesthesia, but scraping the uterine lining is quite painful.

✦ *Endometrial biopsy* is an office procedure and a simplified version of the D&C. A thin tube, called a *cannula*, is inserted through the canal of your cervix, and a tissue sample is obtained by applying suction. Tissue drawn up into the cannula is sent for microscopic evaluation. The cannula is thin enough that dilation of the cervical canal is not necessary. It takes only seconds, but it is still blind and it hurts.

✦ *Hysteroscopy* is the most accurate method to get the job done. The hysteroscope is a multichanneled, thin metal tube with an eyepiece and a light source. When inserted through your cervix into your uterus, a video camera can be attached and your entire uterine cavity shows up on a monitor in full living color. Color prints can be made for future comparison, if needed. Abnormal areas can be easily seen and biopsies, accurately taken. This can be done as an office procedure or as an outpatient hospital procedure if your doctor does not have a hysteroscope. Hysteroscopic tissue sampling is a major step forward in safe and accurate endometrial evaluation. A diagnostic hysteroscopy can be done without anesthesia. If tissue is to be removed, it is painful without anesthesia.

Endometrial cancer can be diagnosed early because it causes abnormal bleeding. With early diagnosis, the cure approaches 100%. It is worth repeating that HRT using both estrogen and progestin does not increase the risk for endometrial cancer. The number of women who die from this disease has declined each year for the past 60 years. If you have abnormal bleeding, whether on HRT or not, discuss it with a knowledgeable physician—NOW!

Breast Cancer

The relationship between breast cancer and HRT is still a cloudy issue. The preponderance of evidence from studies so far shows no increased risk with HRT, but no decrease either (Heinrich 1992). An occasional report out of several dozen shows a link between hormone replacement and breast cancer (Andrews 1992). These are the ones that make headlines in the media of course, so breast cancer fear is never far from the surface of every woman's mind—specially if she is over 40.

A good example of current media coverage was a front page story in the *New York Times* on June 15, 1995, which reported a Harvard study (Nurses' Health Study) showing a 30%–40% increase in breast cancer for women who had used HRT for five years. Buried in the newspaper account were the critical comments of experts in the field, who pointed to flaws in the study and to flaws in the interpretation of the data by the authors. Dr. Trudy Bush, an epidemiologist (researcher who studies large population health trends) at the University of Maryland in Baltimore, commented that the data collected by the Harvard researchers were more consistent with establishing estrogen's role as a cancer *promoter*, rather than as a direct cause of cancer, as the authors had interpreted it and the media had trumpeted it. In other words, estrogen can cause more rapid growth of a breast cancer that is already present, but there is no convincing evidence that it *starts* cancer.

One month after the above story made headlines in all major newspapers and evening TV news shows, another study was published by the University of Washington showing just the opposite results regarding hormone use and breast cancer. The news media were silent. In late 1995, a team of epidemiologists from Wisconsin, Massachusetts, Maine, and New Hampshire published yet another study which again showed no link of long-term hormone use to breast cancer. This study was statistically even more powerful than the others, but the news media again ignored it. I guess good news is no news.

BREAST CANCER STATISTICS

Let us look at the numbers, so you can have some perspective on the size of the problem and the risk. In this decade, approximately 184,000 women in the United States are diagnosed with breast cancer each year, and over 44,000 die from this disease annually. A widely used figure is that one in eight American women who live to age 85 will develop this disease during her lifetime. That is a frightening datum. See Table 7-1 for your chance of developing breast cancer by any given age. Of all the different types of female cancer, 32% of cases are breast cancers, making it the most common. As for cancer deaths, lung cancer has the highest death rate, followed by breast cancer at 18% of all cancer deaths for women (ACOG 1995). That is 10 times higher than the death rate for endometrial cancer, and twice the number of osteoporosis deaths.

The risk of breast cancer increases with age. Nearly 75% of the cases occur in women over age 65, 15% in women under 50, and 6.5% in women under 40. Table 7-1 demonstrates the relationship of aging to the frequency of breast cancer. The media have given considerable publicity to statistics like those in Table 7-1. Women (physicians, too) really believe that one in eight of all American women now living will develop a breast cancer. That is true only if you are talking to a 20-year-old woman who will live to age 85. The table shows that a 60-year-old woman has a nine times greater risk for breast cancer than a 40-year-old ($217 \div 24 = 9$), but a woman who is cancer-free at 60 has only a 1 in 15 chance of developing it if she lives to age 85. That calculation is based on her 1 in 24 lifetime chance of cancer at age 60 minus her 1 in 9 chance at age 85. ($24 - 9 = 15$). That same 60-year-old woman has an 8 in 14 chance of developing heart disease! Any objective observer must concede that heart disease carries a significantly greater risk. I do not want you to feel that I am underplaying breast cancer and the anguish you feel about the prospect of it. I want you to realize that headlines have been misleading the American woman. My interest is in your being presented a balanced picture, so your decisions can be made from a fund of accurate knowledge.

There is another reassuring point about estrogen and breast cancer. Figure 7-1 is a graph from a 1983 study which demonstrates the incidence of female cancers in women who are not taking estrogen. Note that endometrial cancer reaches its peak incidence about the time of menopause and then declines. It has been well established for more than 20 years that unopposed estrogen use is closely linked to endometrial cancer, so it is not surprising that it declines after estrogen production is lost. Now look at the line representing breast cancer. It keeps right on rising into advanced age in spite of the fact that menopause, and estrogen loss, occurred in the early 50s. If estrogen was a factor, the incidence of breast cancer should have declined just as it did with endometrial cancer. This strongly suggests that estrogen as a risk factor is apparently a small one, but the definitive answer is not yet available to us.

Table 7-1	
ODDS OF DEVELOPING BREAST CANCER BY AGE	
By age 25	1 in 19,608
By age 30	1 in 2,525
By age 35	1 in 622
By age 40	1 in 217
By age 45	1 in 93
By age 50	1 in 50
By age 55	1 in 33
By age 60	1 in 24
By age 65	1 in 17
By age 70	1 in 14
By age 75	1 in 11
By age 80	1 in 10
By age 85	1 in 9
Lifetime	1 in 8

Source: National Cancer Institute (1993)

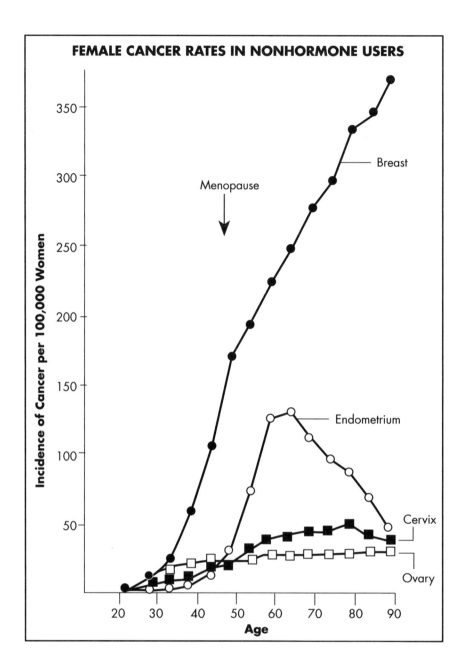

FEMALE CANCER RATES IN NONHORMONE USERS

Menopause

Breast

Endometrium

Cervix

Ovary

Incidence of Cancer per 100,000 Women

Age

Figure 7-1 demonstrates that the two most important risk factors for breast cancer are being a woman, and aging. You probably don't want to stop doing either one of those things.

Epidemiologists point out that the death rate from breast cancer has not significantly changed in 50 years. They also point out that this is in spite of the fact that estrogen has been increasing in use for 40 of those 50 years. If estrogen has been playing a role in breast cancer, it would be reasonable to expect that the death rate would have increased, yet it has not. Epidemiologists have been looking for a causal association between estrogen and breast cancer for five decades and still do not have a definitive answer. The same investigative techniques showed the causal relationship between estrogen and uterine cancer almost 25 years ago, yet the estrogen–breast cancer link has still not been demonstrated by credible studies with statistical power. This suggests that if a causal link exists, it must be in a certain subgroup of women that is too small for current scientific methods to reveal. For the big picture, that is a reassuring inference about estrogen use. However, the death rate has not significantly decreased in 50 years either, reflecting poorly on treatment and prevention.

NEGATIVE SCIENTIFIC STUDIES ON BREAST CANCER AND ESTROGEN USE

Another of the more fearsome studies of recent years came in 1989 from Sweden, where researchers studied 23,244 women over age 35 and reported 10% more breast cancers in women who used combination estrogen-progestin, and 70% more if they used it for over nine years. The news media jumped all over this study too, but later numerous flaws in the study were pointed out, such as: the study was conducted by sending out questionnaires; their results were based on an 11% return, which they used to project their findings to all 23,244. So, in fact, the study was based on a total of 253 breast cancers, which is far too small a number to achieve statistical significance and reach the conclusions they reported. In a follow-up report, the authors corrected their original statistics to reflect that the increased risk was only 1.1 times normal, which is almost the same as for nonusers of estrogen. Plus their data were collected from women who used estradiol valerate, a very potent synthetic estrogen, which is little used in this country. Criticism of this frightening study was not covered by the media.

The conclusion of experts in this field is that more study is definitely needed, because the available evidence is still too limited to convincingly demonstrate either a protective or a detrimental effect of HRT on the risk of breast cancer. Recognized expert doctors like Trudy Bush, Leon Speroff, and Lila Nachtigall recommend that no change be made yet in HRT in our country. They feel that the conflicting results of studies published to date are actually somewhat reassuring, because if a causal connection between estrogen and breast cancer truly existed, the results of all these studies would be in agreement. Contradictory study results mean that if there is any impact of postmenopausal estrogen on breast cancer, it is quite small. Definitive results are anticipated from the Women's Health Initiative (WHI), a randomized clinical trial that is now in progress. WHI will not be completed until about 2005.

NON-NEGATIVE STUDIES ON BREAST CANCER

In 1991, the *Archives of Internal Medicine* reported a meta analysis (an analysis of all 25 previous studies) of women on HRT. It revealed that 21 out of those 25 studies showed little or no increased risk of breast cancer with HRT. Three of the 25 showed a one-and-one-half- to twofold increase, and one, a threefold increase. None of the 25 studies showed an increased number of cancer deaths. This implies that women on HRT are getting diagnosed earlier and therefore enjoying higher cure rates. It is also known that cancer developing in a woman taking HRT is not as aggressive. Cure rates are therefore higher.

Another meta analysis of over 50 studies on estrogen and breast cancer reported the same result of very little causal connection between the two. So, the debate rages on. The evidence is quite strong that estrogen can exaggerate an existing breast cancer, but the evidence does not support claims that it can actually cause a cancer.

RISK FACTORS FOR BREAST CANCER

It is important to point out that while HRT makes all the headlines, there are other risk factors for developing breast cancer. These are much more significant by far than HRT, so you should be familiar with them. Some of them are related to lifestyle influences which you can control; but others, like aging and heredity, are just the way it is. We'll examine each of them.

Family history

Two genes have been identified that can predispose carriers to breast cancer if the genes become mutated. These mutated genes can be passed from carrier to offspring. So far only two are known, but there may be others. Those known are BRCA-1 and BRCA-2, located on chromosomes 17 and 13, respectively. The normal function of these genes is to be a growth suppressor, meaning they limit growth of breast cells. When they undergo a mutation, the ability to suppress cell growth is lost, and the gene is now an oncogene. A cancer may then start if an additional outside influence turns on the oncogene and unrestrained growth is unleashed. It is estimated that 1 in 800 American women carry a mutated BRCA-1 gene. Genetically related breast cancer is thought to account for about 10% of all cases diagnosed.

According to a 1995 study by Shattuck, a woman with a mutated BRCA-1 gene has an 87% lifetime risk for breast cancer and a 63% risk for ovarian cancer.

Each of her children of either gender has a 50% chance of inheriting the mutated gene from her. Males who carry the mutated BRCA-1 gene are at an increased risk of three times for prostate cancer and four times for colon cancer. For carriers of BRCA-2, the lifetime breast cancer risk is 80%, and 20% for ovarian cancer.

If you have a first-degree relative (mother or sister) who has had breast cancer before age 50, or two or more second-degree relatives with breast or ovarian cancer, you should be screened for these mutated genes. DNA testing is complex and expensive. The National Cancer Institute can put you in touch with genetic services at several cancer centers. You or your doctor can acquire more information by calling 1-800-CANCER.

Age

There's nothing you can do about this factor of course. Age is the single most important risk factor for developing breast cancer, as shown in Figure 7-1. More than 75% of breast cancer cases occur after age 50. It should be pointed out that the greatest amount of breast cancer occurs during the part of your life when you have the least estrogen, suggesting that estrogen does not play a major role. Don't forget that Figure 7-1 represents women who do *not* take hormones. The message is to be aware of the fact that aging is a major player, and you should never neglect availing yourself of the screening techniques discussed below.

High fat diet and obesity

Studies have shown that 30% of women with breast cancer are obese and/or consume a diet high in animal fat. Both factors increase your risk by about 50%. For example, fat as a source of calories makes up only 10% to 20% of the traditional Japanese diet—as compared to an average fat intake that is twice as high in the American diet. Among Japanese women, breast cancer occurrences are about 75% lower than those among American women. The fat–breast cancer connection is now being disputed as reported by investigators in the February 8, 1996, *New England Journal of Medicine*. They reviewed seven *cohort* studies, in which similar groups are studied in a prospective manner, proving more reliable than the case control method, a retrospective study of medical records. These seven cohort studies found no evidence of a link between fat intake and breast cancer. The definitive answer will come from a *randomized clinical trial*, the most reliable scientific method in which a study group and a control group are each given a placebo or the test medicine in a randomized fashion—neither the doctor nor the patient knows which is being used. The Women's Health Initiative, mentioned above, will report on the relationship of dietary fat to diseases such as breast cancer. Meanwhile, a low fat diet and avoiding obesity have known benefits in CVD prevention, so please don't abandon the concept.

Alcohol

A large number of studies have produced conflicting results. Most have shown an increased risk of breast cancer with alcohol consumption, but they differ on how much alcohol, how often, and how much more risk. The reasons for this association were unclear in the many studies reported, but the researchers speculate that it has to do with diminished estrogen levels, altered liver function, and adverse effects on DNA in breast cells. The Nurse's Health Study reported in 1987 that perimenopausal women were at four times greater risk with one or more drinks per day than postmenopausal women. By contrast, in 1995 Dr. P. A. Newcomb reported a large study in Massachusetts, Wisconsin, New Hampshire, and Maine on women taking estrogen. They found no significant increase in breast cancer in women who consumed varying amounts of alcohol. The bottom line if you have increased risk factors for breast cancer is to drink only in moderation (one drink per day or less) or abstain.

Smoking

Smoking is a risk not only for your heart, lungs, bones, and skin, but also for your breasts. A 1995 study by Bennicke reported a slight increase in breast cancer for cigarette smokers. It is apparently related to the more than 4,000 toxins, including 16 known carcinogens, in burning tobacco which are thought to cause oncogenic mutations in breast cell genes.

Dr. C. B. Ambrosone and co-workers reported in 1996 that the risk for breast cancer is increased in postmenopausal women who have mutations in an enzyme called *N-acetyltransferase*. This enzyme has important functions in detoxifying (acetylating) carcinogens in tobacco smoke. Postmenopausal women who are slow acetylaters *and* heavy smokers have an increased risk for breast cancer. This was not true for premenopausal women. In the American female population, slow acetylaters make up roughly 65%–90% of women of Middle Eastern descent, 55% of Caucasians, 35% of Blacks, and 10%–20% of Asians. The higher the number of cigarettes smoked and the younger the age at which smoking began, the higher the risk for breast cancer after menopause.

Being a nonsmoker is a really good thing to be.

Exercise

The Harvard Nurses' Health Study found that breast cancer was reduced by 50% for women who exercise about four hours per week. This study was done mostly on perimenopausal women. Postmenopausal women are presently being studied, but the implication is that a sedentary lifestyle may contribute to breast cancer. This benefit was even greater in women who had exercised regularly since their teens and 20s. Now is a good time to get your daughters away from the TV sets and computer keyboards, and maybe you can help them by joining them.

Prior induced abortion

Several studies have shown a small positive association between breast cancer and prior abortions. You may have read about some of them. However, the issue seems to have been laid to rest by a very large European study reported in 1997 by Melbye and coworkers. They reviewed 1.53 million women from government health records and found no association between abortion and breast cancer, even if there had been multiple abortions.

Estrogen exposure from life situations

Prolonged and uninterrupted cyclic estrogen exposure during your life can predispose you to breast cancer. This is especially true in situations where the protective effect of progesterone is absent. Examples are

+ first full-term pregnancy after age 30, or never pregnant. Means more uninterrupted years of monthly estrogen cycles and the accompanying monthly breast changes.
+ early onset of menstrual periods before age 12. More uninterrupted years of estrogen cycles.
+ late menopause after age 54. More lifetime years of estrogen cycles.
+ prolonged perimenopause with anovulation. You lose progesterone's protective anti-estrogen effect if not ovulating.
+ prolonged infertility from anovulation. Progesterone is absent.
+ obesity, meaning more than 20% above ideal body weight. Excess estrogen results from conversion of body fat.
+ if your own birth weight was over 4,000 grams (8 lbs., 8 oz.). Apparently this is related to your fetal exposure to high estrogen levels from your mother (Michels 1996).

"Aha!" you exclaim. "How can you recommend hormone replacement *now*?" Turns out that you can still use HRT, even if the above mentioned risk factors exist for you. Two definitive studies by Kaufman and Wingo have shown that these risks are not magnified if those women use postmenopausal hormone replacement. The issue of hormone replacement and breast cancer will be more thoroughly discussed in Chapter 11.

SCREENING FOR BREAST CANCER

Breast self-examination, physician exams, and mammograms are the bulwark of screening. No laboratory tests yet exist, such as the Pap smear, for breast cancer screening. Screening has been in a ferment in recent years, but a national consensus, which I will explain, seems to be emerging.

Breast self-examination (BSE)

The main advantage of BSE is that after you learn the technique and are doing it on a monthly basis, you become an expert on what your breasts feel like. Any subsequent change in the texture of your breasts will be more readily recognized. Figure 7-2 demonstrates BSE. If you are still menstruating, the best time to do the exam is just after your period has ended. Your breasts are less congested and less tender at this time, and your exam will be more accurate. If you are postmenopausal, just pick a day each month that is easy to remember like the first or the last day.

The drawback of self-examination is that few women feel breast lumps before they are less than a half inch or more in size. This is relatively large. By the time you or your doctor become aware of a mass this size, it may have been present for as much as two years. In view of this fact, a new school of thought is beginning to emerge on the value of BSE. Mammography can detect a lump when it is too small for either you or your doctor to feel. Reliance therefore is shifting more to mammograms than BSE for early detection of breast lumps. More on this below.

Physician breast examination

Even though your doctor's exam suffers limitations for early discovery of breast lumps, a thorough breast exam should be part of any physical examination and gynecologic checkup. If you have concerns about how your breasts feel or doubts about what you are feeling, your doctor's opinion should be solicited. If you are both in agreement that something is suspicious, a mammogram will likely be the next item on the agenda.

Mammography

Screening mammography has been credited for the increase in the breast cancer survival rate from 78% a few years ago to 93% at present. In 1996, Dr. Robert Tarone of the National Cancer Institute's Biostatistics Branch reported a continuing decline in the death rate from breast cancer since 1987. The decline is attributed to earlier diagnosis as the result of screening mammography and improved treatment. This is in spite of the fact that mammograms miss about 10% of new tumors if there are no calcium flecks seen in the tumor mass. Nevertheless, a mammogram can show a lump about a quarter of the size that would be necessary for you or your doctor to detect. Since early detection is crucial to surviving breast cancer, it is increasingly obvious that mammography plays an important role.

A mammogram is done with an X-ray machine that passes radiation through your breasts after they have been compressed to a flatter shape. This can be uncomfortable, so be sure to avoid getting it done during the latter half of your cycle when your breasts are naturally tender. Cancer densities are different

BREAST SELF-EXAMINATION

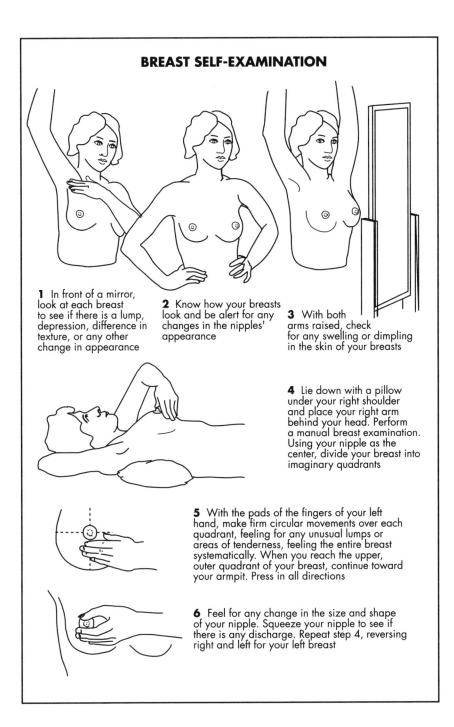

1 In front of a mirror, look at each breast to see if there is a lump, depression, difference in texture, or any other change in appearance

2 Know how your breasts look and be alert for any changes in the nipples' appearance

3 With both arms raised, check for any swelling or dimpling in the skin of your breasts

4 Lie down with a pillow under your right shoulder and place your right arm behind your head. Perform a manual breast examination. Using your nipple as the center, divide your breast into imaginary quadrants

5 With the pads of the fingers of your left hand, make firm circular movements over each quadrant, feeling for any unusual lumps or areas of tenderness, feeling the entire breast systematically. When you reach the upper, outer quadrant of your breast, continue toward your armpit. Press in all directions

6 Feel for any change in the size and shape of your nipple. Squeeze your nipple to see if there is any discharge. Repeat step 4, reversing right and left for your left breast

than others and commonly have tiny calcium deposits that alert the radiologist to their presence. About one in 10 mammograms will find an abnormality that necessitates an additional magnification view for clarification. Sometimes an ultrasound will be needed to distinguish between a fluid filled mass (cyst) and a solid mass. About one-tenth of these follow-up tests lead to a recommendation for a biopsy.

The issue of how often to get a mammogram has been in a state of flux for several years. The original recommendation was to do the first one at age 35, then every two years in your 40s, and annually after 50. Initiating mammography at 35 has now been dropped except in women who are known to be at high risk for breast cancer. In 1993, the National Cancer Institute (NCI) withdrew its recommendation for screening women between 40 and 49, saying that younger breasts triggered too many unnecessary biopsies. The entire scientific community derided this governmental stance and remained firm in the recommendation of a two-year interval. Since then, new evidence has shown that even the recommendation for screening every two years is not sufficient. Leading cancer specialists took strong stands, and now the emerging national consensus is to do annual mammograms on every woman starting at age 40. Medicare historically restricted mammograms for elderly women to every two years, a heartless and disgraceful policy. But on the day in March 1997 when the NCI finally reversed its stance, the president announced to the public that he was directing Medicare to cover annual mammograms on all recipients.

Ultrasound (US)

Ultrasound is nothing more than passage of high frequency sound waves through tissues. It is painless and harmless. Sound waves pass through tissues composed mostly of water but are bounced back if they strike something solid. This creates an image on a monitor, which can be interpreted. It isn't a good primary screening tool for breast cancer because it can't pick up lumps smaller than 1–2 centimeters, and it doesn't distinguish the calcium flecks seen in cancer. It is, however, a useful backup tool for mammography. Ultrasound can distinguish between masses that are cystic (fluid filled) or solid, whereas mammography cannot. A cystic mass may need little more than drainage through a tiny needle, but a solid mass may need a biopsy. It therefore saves a lot of biopsies.

High definition ultrasound imaging

In April 1996, the FDA approved an advanced high definition ultrasound machine designed to tell whether a lump previously detected by mammography, conventional ultrasound, or manual exam is benign or malignant. Studies in several countries with this High Definition Imaging (HDI) machine have shown that it is 99% accurate in predicting noncancerous breast lumps, but only 60% accurate in predicting cancer. In spite of its 40% false positive rate for malignant lumps, HDI will still reduce by 40% the 700,000 breast biopsies being done annually. This will be a definite benefit in reducing the pain, inconvenience, and expense of biopsy diagnosis. HDI will cost up to $300 as compared to a breast biopsy's cost of about $2,500.

Magnetic resonance imaging (MRI)

MRI is not a practical method for primary screening. For one thing, at about $1,600 per exam it is expensive. For another, it is quite a daunting procedure to have done. They roll you into a tube just big enough to accommodate your body. Newer machines use a horseshoe-shaped tube that is not as confining. Then you must lie quite still for half an hour or more while the scan is carried out. The advantages of MRI are the following:

+ it can aid in deciding whether a breast lump is cancerous or not, and possibly avoid a surgical biopsy
+ it can determine whether a cancerous lesion is the sole tumor or in multiple locations. This will aid in the decision of whether surgery can be a lumpectomy or a mastectomy
+ it uses no radiation

A disadvantage of MRI is that it may identify lumps that are not cancerous, leading to needless biopsies.

Positive emission tomography (PET)

This is a scanning device which measures uptake of radioactive sugar by cancerous breast tumors. Cancer cells have a higher metabolic rate than normal cell, so they need more sugar to keep going. They take up more of the radioactive sugar than normal cells, and this shows readily on the scan as a "hot spot." The National Cancer Institute has funded a study to see if PET can identify cancer cells in lymph glands of the armpit. If this proves to be a reliable technique, it will save a lot of painful surgery in women with proven breast cancer.

Genetic screening

This new technology was mentioned earlier. Since 90% of breast cancer is not hereditary, this will not be widely used. In those women who have a strong family history of breast and ovarian cancer, however, knowledge of having a mutated BRCA-1 gene can pose some weighty problems. Think about some of the medical, ethical, legal, and moral issues involved if a cancer-free woman knows she has more than an 80% chance of future breast cancer, and 50%–60%

chance of ovarian cancer. Must the potential for future disease be disclosed if it becomes known? Who else has a right to this information: a husband? a fiancé? an employer? your insurance company? your children? the bank where you are applying for a 30-year loan? Other questions are: should your breasts be removed? your ovaries too? An avalanche of genetic information such as this is about to descend upon us. Our wisdom will be sorely tried, but talented people are already working on guidelines for genetic screening of breast cancer and how to handle the information it might disclose.

CAN PROGESTIN HELP?

There has been a growing interest in whether progestin may be protective against breast cancer. It is based on the fact that in the uterine endometrium, progestin depletes the number of available estrogen receptors, thereby protecting from cancer. The logical expectation is that it should do the same in breast tissue. Only two studies in the early and mid-1980s support this logic (Gambrell 1983 and WHO 1984). The Harvard study referred to above reported in June 1995 that they found no evidence that progestin was protective in breast tissue. Other studies are under way in the Women's Health Initiative, and we breathlessly await their results.

Other Cancers and Hormone Use

Not much is published on the relationship between HRT and other cancers. An early 1995 report by an epidemiologist with the American Cancer Society, Dr. Eugenia Calle, indicated that women who have used hormone replacement have a significant decrease in colon cancer. She reported on 422,373 women between age 45 and 70 who were followed for seven years. Those on HRT had a 45% decreased risk of death from colon cancer. This jumped to a 55% decrease if they had been on HRT for 10 years or more. Such a study must await confirmation by other researchers to give it general acceptance, but this is a potential bombshell of good news for the third most common female cancer.

Oral contraceptives reduce the risk of ovarian cancer by 80% (Harkinson 1992). More than a dozen studies of HRT and ovarian cancer have failed to demonstrate any causal link. The problem, however, is that ovarian cancer is not common (15 per 100,000 women per year), and the studies never have large enough numbers for the results to reach statistical significance.

Hormone replacement plays no role in lung cancer, which is your number one cancer risk, and no role in cervical cancer.

Summing Up

I most fervently wish I could say to you that HRT poses no particular risk for you with respect to breast cancer. This would be a much shorter chapter if that were true. I hear your concern and I understand your anguish. Dr. Leon Speroff feels it is appropriate to say that there is a small concern that long-term estrogen use *could* be associated with an increased risk. At the present time, however, there is no definitive evidence that the standard hormone doses used for CVD prevention and osteoporosis prevention are linked to an increased risk of breast cancer. The odds favor HRT's safety, but you may still feel that you just can't bet the farm on it. Perhaps it will help your internal debate to consider that the odds of your living a longer and healthier life are much more enhanced by prevention of heart disease, a five- to tenfold greater risk than breast cancer. This was my wife's decision.

All of the foregoing neither exonerates estrogen's role, if any, in breast cancer nor nails estrogen to the wall as the culprit. At this stage of knowledge, or lack of it, your decision must be based on whether you feel the benefit of HRT outweighs the risk. CVD protection, osteoporosis prevention, and symptom improvement should be on one side of the scale, and cancer risk plus hormone side effects, on the other. The statistics show that your life expectancy is much greater if you *do* use HRT, but the decision must still be within your own personal comfort zone for the level of risk you can accept.

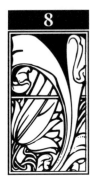

VISIBLE CHANGES
FEMININITY'S SPOILSPORTS

Skin, breasts, vaginas, vulvas, muscles, veins, and hair growth are the topics of this chapter. Although far from a fatal subject, visible changes in appearance can cause a lot of anguish for many. A discussion of what happens, and what you can do about what happens, follows.

Atrophy means the failure to grow, or the wasting away, of tissue because of inadequate cellular nutrition. Atrophic changes in many parts of your body are part of the natural process of aging. In many cases they are the result of diminishing blood flow. Some atrophic problems are remediable; with others, the best you can do is slow it down. So far, the aging process is an unstoppable juggernaut that no one has defeated. This publication makes no claim of victory either, *but* I've got some moves for you.

Atrophic skin, atrophic breasts, and atrophic vaginas are major strikes against major features of a woman's body. You place a great store of value on these areas, as do your men and our culture. More value than should be assigned, perhaps, but there it is. There is a lot more to femininity and being a woman than smooth skin, firm breasts, and a functioning vagina, of course; however, their removal from the overall picture is too often a severe blow to a woman's self esteem. If it isn't a severe, or even a mild blow for you, feel free to skip on to the discussion of sex at midlife in Chapters 9 and 10. For those remaining, let us press on.

Skin

Your skin is the biggest organ you've got. It has two layers: *epidermis* (what you see) and *dermis* (inner layer), and beneath these is the *subdermis* (fatty layer under the dermis). Skin is normally very pliable and elastic because of connective tissues called *collagen* and *elastin*. Aging of skin and wrinkling occur when production of these two connective tissues declines or when they themselves deteriorate. The result is, you guessed it, WRINKLES.

WHAT CAUSES SUCH AN OUTRAGE?

Genes are part of it. Aging in cells throughout your body appears to be genetically programmed at birth. Each of your trillions of cells has DNA strands in its nucleus on which genes are located. The genes control a variety of cellular metabolic activities including how frequently the cell will reproduce itself and how long the cell will live. For skin cells, life lasts about one month. As aging occurs, the genetic messages are gradually changed. There is diminished hormone production, as well as decreased production of the nearly three dozen growth factors necessary for new cell formation. Cells throughout your body slow down in their frequency of division into new cells. So, aging of your skin is part of "planned obsolescence" that you have had from the start of life.

Menopause and low estrogen levels also play a role in wrinkling and dry skin. Estrogen receptors exist in skin, especially in the facial skin. A reduction in estrogen production is coincident with thinning of skin, a well established fact. Collagen is known to decrease about 1% per year after age 25, but this increases to 2% per year after menopause. When HRT is begun, the dermis plumps up and skin thickens again as collagen production increases. Wrinkles lessen slightly with this treatment, but HRT is no fountain of youth in this regard. By age 60, HRT users have thinning of their skin, although it is still about twice the skin thickness as that of nonusers.

Ultraviolet radiation (UV light) from sunlight is *the* major contributor to skin aging. The term for this is *photoaging*. It is caused by the release of free radicals in your skin cells from UV exposure. Free radicals are unstable molecules that go zooming about bumping into and damaging cell membranes. They can cause damage anywhere in the body, but in skin, the effect may be dramatic with wrinkling, sagging, and a mottled pigmentation. Controlling the effects involves skin protection: Sunblock creams with a sun protection factor (SPF) rating of 15 or more are effective. Make sure to put the sunblock on 30 minutes before sun exposure, so it will bond to your skin. Protective clothing is beneficial and, naturally, avoiding sunlight exposure always works. Sunlight protection becomes very important after 40 because melanin in your skin decreases, and burning, with skin damage, is much more likely. Perimenopausal and postmenopausal suntans are *not* cool.

Cigarette smoking causes wrinkling of the skin earlier and more severely, depending on how heavily you smoke. Toxins in cigarette smoke are thought to damage small blood vessels that nourish skin. Smoking also decreases estrogen production, which can cause premature aging. Cigarette smokers in their 40s often have wrinkling as severe as women 20 years older. Characteristic smoker-wrinkles are deep smile lines around the eyes and radial wrinkles about the lips.

Your skin likes for your diet to be balanced. This means a diet rich in fruits, vegetables, whole grains, and complex carbohydrates. The concept of what constitutes a balanced diet is covered in Chapter 14. The myth that a high animal fat intake is good for your skin is not true (Fulton 1996). The exception is in chronic dieters with inadequate fat and protein intake. They often have dry skin.

A healthy and smoother skin is also dependent on your consuming about two quarts of fluid each day. This maintains the plumpness of your skin. On the flip side, alcohol dehydrates your skin, so this should not be a significant part of your daily two-quart fluid intake.

Drug abuse is a skin abuser. Not only does it age you faster, but you will appear drawn and haggard as your aging progresses.

Regular exercise stimulates blood flow and transports nutrients to your skin. Many dermatologists feel that vigorous exercise is more effective for a vibrant appearing skin than any of the huge array of cosmetic products now available for this purpose.

OK, SO WHAT'S TO BE DONE?

Daily facial care must be consistent. Good facial skin care can be achieved in only a few minutes each day. It is not necessary to cleanse your face each morning if you have done so before retiring the night before. Just stimulate your skin with a cold washcloth and pat dry. Then apply a moisturizer and put on your makeup if you wear it. During the rest of the day, no special care is needed. Don't forget a sunblock before putting on your makeup if you will be out of doors. In the evening, use a cleanser or a makeup-removing cleanser, apply a toner if you have oily skin, and finally use a moisturizer before going to bed.

Daily hand care is important because for most women, hands take a beating. If you wash them frequently or they are often wet during the day, the consequence is dry hands. For washing, Dove and Neutragena, the transparent soap, are mild cleansers that are well tolerated. If a hand cream is applied every time you wash, improvement in your dry hands will be evident in just a few days. Keep some handy at all of your sinks. At night apply a moisturizer before you climb into bed. If you have those irregular brown pigmented areas called "liver spots," glycolic acid–laced moisturizers will help, as long as you use a sunscreen along with it when outside. The first step in helping liver spots is to get sun protection.

Daily body care is simple and easy. We tend to overwash in our country. Taking a bath, especially a long hot soak, dries out your skin. In the winter when the weather is cold and blustery, and heating systems are turned up, your skin will be much drier. Showering or bathing will only add to dryness. A shower every other day with a sponge bath in between will usually suffice for cleanliness and keep drying to a minimum. For a cleanser, Dove and Neutragena are mild, cleanse well, and are not drying. During your shower, a loofah sponge used vigorously from your neck down will help remove dry and dead cells from your skin surface. It is quite invigorating, as it increases circulation of blood and tones your skin. After your bath or shower, pat your body dry and use a moisturizer all over, including your feet, while still slightly damp. This helps retain the moisture in your skin.

DAMAGE REPAIR

If you already have wrinkles and other skin changes, cosmetic surgery can be considered. An amazing variety of surgical procedures can help. These include face lift, forehead lift, eyelid lift, neck lift, and tummy tuck. The operations utilize liposuction, laser resurfacing, and newer surgical approaches with endoscopes. Endoscopes are multichanneled tubes that are inserted through tiny incisions. Surgical instruments are passed through the channels, and a video camera is attached to view the operation on a monitor. Cosmetic surgery can be remarkably effective (and expensive), but nonsurgical treatments such as the following are also available.

+ *Dermabrasion* is an outpatient procedure utilizing high-speed brushes to remove epidermal and dermal tissue from fine wrinkles. It is then replaced with new skin. The result is permanent. Dermatologists and plastic surgeons do these procedures.
+ *Chemical peels* are also outpatient procedures to remove fine wrinkles with permanent result. Some estheticians do minor peels, but deep peels should be done by dermatologists or plastic surgeons.
+ *Retin-A* is a vitamin A derivative in a cream used for fine to moderate wrinkles in women age 50 to 70. It does not work for everyone and may be very overrated. A related drug called *tretinoin*, and marketed as Renova, has been approved by the FDA for use before sunlight exposure to prevent wrinkles.
+ *Collagen injections* are placed in the skin. They fill out deep wrinkles, like smile lines around eyes and laugh lines around the mouth. It does a good job, but needs to be repeated about every 6–9 months.
+ *Cosmetic laser treatments* are coming into greater use. Laser light vaporizes the surface layer of skin cells, which reduces or eliminates age lines. Skin resurfacing with the laser requires anesthesia and results in painful, red skin for about a month. Dermatologists and plastic surgeons should be consulted.

Other than these specialized, nonsurgical treatments, the other most effective steps to be taken have already been mentioned: cleanse gently and moisturize. When you wash, use a nonsoap cleanser and warm water; this way they won't eliminate the natural oil barrier that keeps your skin moist. Apply skin moisturizer immediately after your skin has been hydrated (bath, shower) to reduce water loss. Any kind of oil or greasy product will do nicely, like petroleum jelly, vegetable shortening, or any oil-based ointment or cream. Use oil-based cosmetics, and avoid the drying effect of perfumed skin products. Use a humidifier in your home if you live in a dry climate. Drink plenty of water, which is good for your body and your skin. Skin requires about two quarts of fluids each day to remain hydrated. Finally, minimize dehydrating agents such as caffeine, alcohol, diuretics, saunas, and dry air.

Breasts

Breasts have been the subject of such romanticism, flights of fancy, and adoration in our culture and its art and literature over the centuries that they

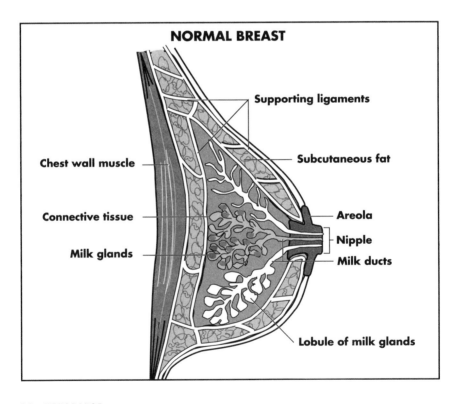

NORMAL BREAST

often become related with a woman's very femininity. Small wonder, the dismay, then, that may be provoked by changes during the middle years.

ANATOMY

Breasts are mostly composed of glands (alveoli) where milk is produced, and the alveoli are then connected to the nipple by ducts. These structures are surrounded by fat, and the whole arrangement is contained in skin and supported by ligaments (Cooper's ligaments) attached to the chest wall. Figure 8-1 shows the anatomy of the breast. Alveoli and ducts are very sensitive to hormonal influence. They become thicker in the last half of each menstrual cycle when estrogen and progesterone production is high. Breasts are then fuller, and often tender, as you well know.

THE MENOPAUSAL EFFECT

When estrogen and progesterone production declines with perimenopause and menopause, breast tissues become atrophic. Cooper's ligaments lose their elasticity. As a result, breasts shrink in size and sag lower on the chest wall. This is particularly true in thin women. In obese women, the shrunken breast tissue tends to be replaced with fat. Nipples may get flatter and lose their erectile ability. Pointing forward goes to pointing downward.

"Not fair!" you exclaim. Well then, what is to be done? Don't look to hormone replacement for much help. Breasts get a little more firm for some women using HRT, but Cooper's ligaments do not get any shorter so sagging is not reversed. However, some new engineering marvels in bra design have emerged, with the potential for a great deal of help. Cosmetic breast surgery has been popularized in recent years, but it is expensive and is not trouble free. So, there isn't any magic remedy for midlife breast change.

My own opinion is that with the continuing emergence of new midlife sexual role models, our culture will accept midlife breast changes as they are. You can then be comfortable with the fact that there is more to femininity than the body type that our culture has prescribed for you thus far.

Vaginas and Vulvas

Vaginas and vulvas are lined with, and covered with, skin. It should come as no surprise, therefore, that they suffer the same atrophic vagaries as skin elsewhere on your body. Figure 8-2 is a representation of normal vulvar anatomy. Visual changes in your vagina and vulva do occur, but the more important change is functional, with all the secondary ripple effects of altered sexuality.

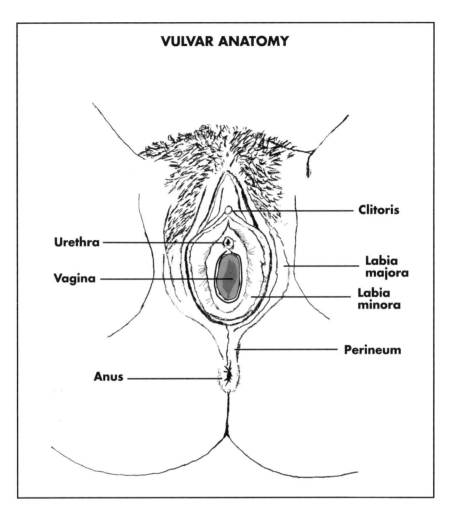

VULVAR ANATOMY

Clitoris

Urethra

Vagina

Labia majora

Labia minora

Perineum

Anus

Vaginal tissues are *very* hormone sensitive and their response to falling estrogen levels is dramatic. Vessels bringing blood to the vaginal lining shrink, which decreases normal nutrition and causes loss of collagen. Just as in skin elsewhere, this results in atrophy. The vaginal lining becomes thin and pale and loses its elasticity. Prolonged vaginal atrophy leads to vaginal *stenosis*, a shrinking of the diameter and length of the vagina, to the point that sex may not be possible. The pH (acidity) in your vagina is normally 4.5 or lower; it rises to over 4.5 when it is atrophic. The changed acidity leads to irritation, discharge, and a greater susceptibility to infection. With diminished blood flow, vaginal lubrication is less, and a feeling of dryness occurs.

Atrophic changes in the vulva outside the vagina result from collagen loss here, too. These are manifested as shrinking of the labia majora (outer hair-bearing folds), shrinking of the labia minora (innermost folds), loss of hair, and dryness. Atrophic vulvar skin is commonly very itchy too. These changes do not happen suddenly, but when dryness, irritation, and loss of elasticity are all present at the same time, sex becomes painful. This uncomfortable situation is known as *dyspareunia* by doctors, but everyone else calls it *awful*. Negative sexual experiences usually cause decreased sexual desire, anxiety, loss of self-esteem, and damaged relationships. Prevention is a much better plan. See below.

Bladder and urethral atrophy also occurs from collagen loss. Both structures are derived from the same tissues as is the vagina, making them estrogen sensitive. The common result of atrophy is a burning sensation during urination (dysuria), an increased need to urinate (urge incontinence), and involuntary loss of urine with pressure as from sneezing, coughing, or laughing (stress incontinence). Estrogen loss with diminished collagen contributes to *cystocele* (sagging of the bladder), *rectocele* (sagging rectum), and *uterine prolapse* (sagging uterus). Any of these latter three conditions can contribute to urinary incontinence. In the past, it had been thought that HRT did not benefit these three conditions. Dr. Daniel Mishell, professor and chairman of Ob/Gyn at the University of Southern California, disagrees. He finds that using vaginal estrogen restores the lost collagen to the extent that the need for surgical procedures to correct these conditions is diminished (Mishell 1995). In 1994, the Swedish government approved a nonprescription 10 microgram estradiol vaginal pellet, after it was determined that its use would save their health care system $200 million annually in treatment costs for the above conditions. A negative note in this regard was sounded by Dr. J. A. Fantl and coworkers in a 1994 report that studied 83 women with urinary incontinence. They found no improvement in urinary symptoms, suggesting that estrogen does not restore lost tone in the supporting structures of the bladder, urethra, and vagina. So, there is no general agreement on this point, but most observers do agree that estrogen use prior to surgery will expedite healing from the operation.

PREVENTION AND TREATMENT OF GENITOURINARY ATROPHY

Painful sex and altered urinary function have a dramatic negative effect on the ease and quality of sexuality for couples. This makes prevention, or successful treatment, extremely important. Estrogen replacement is invariably successful in relieving these atrophic tissue symptoms: Relief for painful sex is evident in about a month, if the problem has not been present for too long; urinary symptom relief requires six to 12 months, so be patient and give it a chance if you opt for HRT.

Other measures, some of them available over the counter, can be helpful. (The first two are not really to be found at your local pharmacy.)

◆ Sexual excitement itself causes increased blood flow and improves lubrication of your vaginal lining. Any form of sexual activity about twice a week, including self-stimulation, helps keep your vagina healthy even if you don't take hormones. So the word is keep on keepin' on.

◆ Slow down. Younger women may get sexual lubrication in only a minute or so of stimulation, whereas postmenopausal women may require as much as 15 minutes or more. Let your partner know this and proceed at a more measured pace, which is more fun anyhow.

◆ Lubricants. If no amount of time is going to get you wet, go for a lubricant. Saliva works great although there is a limited duration of effect because of rapid drying. K-Y Jelly and Astroglide last longer, are really slick, and wash away easily since they are water soluble. Petroleum jelly lasts longer still, but it is not water soluble so cleanup is messy. Also, petroleum jelly can weaken latex condoms, so be careful! A newer brand of vaginal moisturizer called Replens is also effective because it lowers the vaginal pH. This results in more natural lubrication, and it lasts for two to three days. This does not mean you must have sex continuously for three days if you use Replens of course (Imagine!), only that you do not have to apply it every time just before sex.

◆ Estrogen vaginal cream works wonders for an atrophic vagina in restoring the lost elasticity, moisture, and proper pH. Estrogen is absorbed into your bloodstream this way though, so caution is needed here if you are someone who must not take estrogen, like certain cancer patients. In addition to *your* bloodstream, it gets into *his* bloodstream too through the skin of his penis and urethra. Do not use estrogen vaginal cream as a sexual lubricant. One report has been published about male breast enlargement from this source, so I suppose if he switches to soprano and starts wearing bras, you might just want to cut back a bit on that cream. An even better product for vaginal estrogen replacement, called Estring, was marketed in 1997. It is an estrogen-containing device much like a diaphragm ring. You insert it into your vagina and get a slow, steady release of estrogen. It lasts three months. Small amounts of estrogen get into your circulation, but not enough so that unopposed estrogen precautions are necessary.

Muscles

A steady reduction in muscular strength is distressingly common as aging progresses. This is atrophy at work again. Height, weight, and the level of physical activity are important factors affecting muscular atrophy. When muscular competence declines, postmenopausal women are subject to all the hazards of slips, slides, and falls, with their attendant injuries, and life-threatening disabilities. This is particularly true for severely osteoporotic women and their devastating fractures. Keeping physically active is, therefore, crucially important.

Women using HRT do not experience this age-related muscular atrophy, as demonstrated by a handgrip test in a 1987 study by Dr. J. A. Cauley. The obvious HRT advantage here is not only the prevention of fractures, but also the preservation of the *ability* to exercise. This keeps your muscles supple and your balance intact, and both of these aid in preventing falls. Exercise will be covered more extensively in Chapter 14.

Varicose Veins

Varicose veins appear on your legs and slowly worsen as skin elasticity declines. They can be recognized by their serpentine configuration and by how they stand out from the skin surface. They are distinctly different from spider veins, which are generally flat to the surface, red or blue in color, and multibranched. I'll get to spider veins in a minute.

VEIN ANATOMY

Veins are the vessels that return blood to the heart. They have one-way valves, allowing blood to flow toward the heart but preventing backflow. However, when veins dilate, the valves fail, allowing backward flow of blood between heartbeats. Called a varicosity, this occurrence has caused the vein to bulge permanently.

WHO GETS THEM

Women who are genetically predisposed are at a greater risk of getting varicose veins during hormone changes in pregnancy and, in some, even with birth control pills. Prolonged standing on the job, tight fitting garments (garters, knee highs), being overweight, and a sedentary lifestyle all can contribute. Some think that crossing your legs is a cause because of increased vein pressure. On a preventive note, newer types of knee highs are now available that do not constrict at the top, so they would be an acceptable choice when shopping for socks.

WHY WORRY?

The major health risk of varicose veins is that occasionally an inflammatory condition called phlebitis occurs with clotting in a varicose vein. Rarely, a portion of the clot can break loose and travel to your lungs (pulmonary embolism), and this is a major health and/or life threat.

WHAT CAN I DO?

Treatment of varicose veins can be the surgical removal of them (vein stripping) and the surgical ligation of them (tying off the vein) so that the blood is rerouted through other vessels. Multiple small incisions are usually necessary and, of course, leave multiple small scars. Nonsurgical management can often be accomplished by wearing support stockings or support panty hose. These garments do not reverse the varicosities, but they help prevent aching associated with standing.

SPIDER VEINS

Spider veins, also partly hereditary, are dilated veins near the surface of the skin. They pose no health threat. They appear between ages 30 and 50 and are associated with standing jobs, pregnancy, direct trauma, and varicose veins. Treatment can be *sclerotherapy*, which is the injection of an irritant into the vein, causing blood flow to stop. *Electrodesiccation* can work also. Here, tiny needles carrying electric current are used to damage the vein and stop blood flow. Cosmetic laser treatment of spider veins is more widespread, and more effective than many other methods. Application of cosmetics works for some. Tattooing the skin has been tried but with limited success. None of these treatments will prevent additional spider veins from occurring, so whatever you elect to do is going to be an ongoing process.

Hair Growth

Hair changes in postmenopausal women can involve too much hair, called *hirsutism*, or too little, *alopecia*. Excessive hair growth is typically on the face, upper lip, nipples, chest, lower back, and lower abdomen. Some women just have more hair than others as their normal body compliment. What we are talking about here is more hair than you had.

HIRSUTISM

Too much hair can be associated with use of certain drugs like Dilantin (for convulsive disorders), Minoxidil (for severe high blood pressure), Proglycem (for hypoglycemia), testosterone (commonly used in menopause), and anabolic steroids used by muscle builders. The most common cause of increased hair is the male hormone *testosterone*. This hormone is secreted by both sexes, just as is estrogen. The difference is that in your gender, only tiny amounts of testosterone are produced, both in the ovaries and the adrenal glands. Usually the tiny amounts of testosterone can never make any difference because of the huge opposing amounts of estrogen that you produce. After menopause however, estrogen is dramatically reduced by 80%–90%; testosterone, on the other hand, is only about halved in amount. Testosterone then can start doing malelike things, such as growing hair. There isn't enough of it to turn you into a Sylvester Stallone, but it can make you more hairy.

If you really get a lot of new hair, check with your doctor because certain types of tumors (both benign and malignant) can have the same effect. Hirsutism is a common accompaniment of Cushing's syndrome in which the adrenal glands produce excessive amounts of cortisol. Women with polycystic ovarian syndrome produce more testosterone than normal and grow more hair. Insulin resistance is common with aging, which leads to higher insulin levels, and this is associated with higher testosterone production too. The same is true for obesity.

GET RID OF UNSIGHTLY HAIR

To get rid of unsightly hair, you can use a depilatory, bleach it, destroy it with electrolysis, shave it, use a waxing preparation, or get cosmetic laser treatment. (By the way, shaving does not make it grow back faster.) In perimenopausal women, low dose birth control pills are helpful because they slow down ovarian function by reducing FSH and LH stimulation of the ovaries. You get plenty of female hormone, but less testosterone. In postmenopausal women, HRT serves the same purpose. Aldactone (spironolactone) is a diuretic drug that has antitestosterone properties. It may be prescribed for hirsutism but can produce disagreeable side effects such as irregular periods, fatigue, nausea, and headaches.

ALOPECIA

As for loss of hair, it is quite usual for women over 50 to experience thinning of the hair. Normally you lose about 75 hairs each day, and up to four times that many after a shampoo. Actual balding or malelike temporal loss is quite rare. If this happens, it should be investigated for other potentially more serious causes. Bleaches, coloring, straightening, and permanents can chemically damage hair, so it breaks off easily. This is not permanent, of course, and may be reduced or prevented by a protein hair conditioner after shampooing. Direct hair trauma and breaking of hair shafts may occur with braids, pony tails, curlers, elastic hair bands, and too much teasing.

Other conditions and situations associated with hair loss include

✦ various drugs such as amphetamines, antidepressants, anticonvulsants, lithium, and chemotherapy for certain cancers
✦ a sudden and severe stress, even if it was as long as six months ago
✦ high fever
✦ sudden weight loss from a crash diet
✦ poor nutrition, especially if deficient in iron
✦ prolonged general anesthesia
✦ certain thyroid or pituitary gland problems
✦ chronic illnesses such as kidney or liver failure, cancer, diabetes, Hodgkin's disease, and systemic lupus erythematosis

Estrogen will help slow the thinning of scalp hair after menopause and may thicken it slightly. For some women, the thinning is genetic, and HRT does not have much to offer. Minoxidil, marketed as Rogaine, is a nonprescription drug that has been approved for treatment of "male-pattern baldness." It works, but only so long as you keep applying it to your scalp twice each day.

Summing Up

This has been a chapter about visible bodily changes that may affect you during your transition to menopause. They may be bothersome but, on the other hand, not troubling. Fortunately, if some of these changes are troubling to you, there are effective remedies available.

Genitourinary atrophy (vagina, vulva, bladder, and urethra) produces significant symptoms that deserve serious consideration. Painful sex for *you* is bad enough, but it can also adversely affect your partner's sexual performance if he is aware that intercourse is painful for you. Both of your sex drives may become depressed, sex may stop, and neither of you may care. A loving couple may drift apart because of a preventable problem. These and other atrophic changes of the aging process, if viewed negatively, may lead to unwelcome problems with self-esteem and quality of life for both of you. It is much better for the two of you to understand what is happening and to talk about it with each other, with peers, and with your health adviser. Then, after you have made an informed decision, proceed with your plan of management.

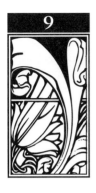

9

SEX AFTER MENOPAUSE

CHANGED, BUT ALIVE AND WELL

Here we will discuss the effects that cultural and personal attitudes have on sex in menopausal women. You will learn how estrogen loss causes both anatomic and functional change. Resolution of personal and partnership problems is emphasized. Techniques for successfully dealing with the changes you might experience are covered.

Biologically, menopause represents the completion of reproductive ability and the end of menstrual periods, but it certainly does *not* signal the end of sexuality. During the transition phase of perimenopause through menopause, when all of the physical and emotional changes are in progress, many of you are so distracted by these events that a blunting of sexual desire may occur. Upon emerging from the transition, however, and with the help of various modalities to be discussed, sexuality remains intact for the large majority of women.

By this time in your life, the kids may be off and running, career goals may have been accomplished, and there is less stress in everyday life. An opportunity to reexplore sex in new and different ways presents itself. The wild and steamy sex of youth will not likely recur, but with maturation of both partners, a deeper intimacy is possible. The wisdom of years makes it more likely that you and your partner will appreciate that sex is a relationship event, rather than simply an urge to be gratified. Women have always known this. And although true that physiologic and anatomic genital changes occur with menopause that can have an adverse impact on good sex, you and your partner will no doubt come to find that the most significant influence on sexuality comes from the most important sex organ of all—your brain.

Attitudes about Midlife

American women generally regard midlife as an unattractive stage. It is hardly surprising when you consider how you have been bombarded all of your life by a youth-oriented mass media bias and by the rigid definition of feminine beauty our culture imposes. At age 50, you obviously don't look like you did 25 years before, so worry and doubt about physical attractiveness is common. This quickly translates to worry and doubt about sexual attractiveness. Worry about almost anything can have a withering effect on sexual enjoyment.

Contributing to the problem is the fact that not enough sexual role models exist for midlife women as yet. This is changing, however, and the change is occurring at an accelerating rate as the boomer generation, with its energy and imagination, moves further into the perimenopausal-postmenopausal era. Model/actress Lauren Hutton is reported to have said she could accept having her 20-year-old body again, but not without her 50-year-old brain.

More women are achieving success in fields that Americans consider important such as business, industry, arts, entertainment, politics, and the professions. Men have long enjoyed high regard for accomplishment in these fields. What is under way now is not a role reversal for the genders, but a sea change for *women* that will indeed provide midlife role models. It will dramatically reduce for most, and eliminate for many, the concerns women have about midlife attractiveness and, in turn, sexuality.

Dr. Gloria Bachman's study at the Robert Wood Johnson Medical School in New Jersey showed that 35% of women experience decreased sexual desire after menopause. This means that 65% do not, so perhaps you won't have a problem at all. A Danish study found that 9% of women reported their sexuality was *enhanced* postmenopausally (Koster 1991). "Well, those are mighty encouraging words," you may interject, "but I *do* have a problem . . . *now*, so let's talk about it."

OK, SO LET'S TALK ABOUT IT

If the above statement is true of you, then you have already taken the first of three steps necessary to resolving it: You have recognized that a problem exists. Changes have taken place in your body and in your sexuality that concern you. For women whose sexual experiences have never been satisfactory, menopause can represent the opportune time to abandon sex and step out of the arena altogether. On the other hand, if you desire improved sex and deeper intimacy, you are well advised to do something about it now. The longer such a problem persists after menopause, the more difficult it becomes to resolve. The physical changes can be easily and reliably improved with estrogen. If they have persisted so long as to generate deep emotional reactions and a negative attitude toward sex, this complication makes it much more difficult to deal with successfully. The take-home message: Don't delay acknowledging your problem with sex.

The second step is to seek help from someone knowledgeable about your problem. If your sexual desire has plummeted since hot flashes started, fatigue has overwhelmed you, vaginal dryness has made sex painful, your moods have been gyrating wildly, and you haven't been able to find the blasted car keys—if all that and more has been on your plate, then a consultation is in order. It should be with a physician who understands menopause and can fairly present the various options available to you. It can be your family practitioner, an internist, a gynecologist, or a specialist in a menopause clinic. On the other hand, if your sexual desire is depressed because you perceive yourself as sexually undesirable and this has persisted for many years, your partner doesn't bring you flowers anymore, sex is about as exciting as watching paint dry, you are faking orgasms because he is faking foreplay, and neither of you gives a darn—that's a load. In this type of case, a consultation with a psychologist, a marriage counselor, or a sex therapist would be advisable. In today's health care system, you may need to start with your primary care physician and then seek secondary care on their referral. A recommendation for a sex counselor in your area may be obtained by contacting the

American Association of Sex Educators, Counselors, and Therapists
435 North Michigan Avenue, Suite 1717
Chicago, IL 60611
(312) 644-0828

Step three is communication. For most of us, this is difficult. It is not hard to talk about sex as it relates to other people, but it sure is if it's about your sexual relationship. The sexual revolution was launched by the flower children during the age of Aquarius over 30 years ago. Since then, we may have been talking more about sex in nearly any sphere of our culture you can name, but we have not been communicating well at all. We sidestepped or muted things that are truly important: personal sexual preferences, the love part of the equation, and the importance of fidelity, to name but three.

So, now you have recognized you have a problem, you have sought help from a knowledgeable source, but you feel like a fish out of water when it comes to talking about it. Nevertheless, *do* talk about it. It is well documented that simply discussing sex can do more to relieve the problem than sophisticated psychotherapy (Edelman 1992). This finding suggests that you and your partner can make some inroads and perhaps bypass third-party help. To achieve this, the two of you need to be a receptive, nonjudgmental, and sensitive audience for each other. If you find that too difficult, get help. The goals of effective communication, as advocated by psychologist Dr. Mardell Grothe are

- to enroll your partner as a fellow problem solver in your particular situation. This promotes cooperation, a sense of satisfaction, and ensures an intimacy between the two of you that usually comes out of any mutual effort.
- to find out what your partner's needs are. You already know what yours are, and you know that your needs are not being met. Still, find out what his are because if you make that effort, he is much more likely to be sensitive and inquisitive to yours.
- to be nonconfrontational. "I fake orgasm because you fake foreplay." *Now* you are arguing. Make your partner feel safe in talking to you, because talking will relieve anxiety and dispel misconceptions. At some point you do need to state your needs, because unstated needs are usually unmet needs. Better to say, "I want our sex life to satisfy us both." Now you can talk.
- to make it a dialogue as opposed to a lecture. The topic you wish to discuss, and the problem you wish to resolve should be regarded as a process, not a single event. If the time or the place or the situation is not right for resolution of your differences, then table the discussion. In the near future, a more appropriate time should be found. Talking about sex makes most people feel uncomfortable, but keep in mind that sex itself may not be the central issue. It could well be that you and your partner need to feel that each of you is satisfying the other's need for caring, respect, and intimacy. You need to give yourself permission to change, and your partner needs to give it also. Getting those issues satisfied can lead to great sex.

Sexual Anatomy Changes and Sexual Response Changes

Anatomic and physiologic changes are the two major categories of observable change that influence sexuality at menopause. It is not hard to imagine that sexual organ changes are closely related to physiologic response. If your vagina has lost its elasticity making sex painful, then your sexual response is not likely to be one of wild and thrashing orgasms.

CHANGES IN RESPONSE

First let's look at *physiologic sexual response changes*. For a response to have any chance of getting under way, it usually needs to be preceded by sexual interest. Sexual interest may be influenced negatively in a great variety of ways at midlife: boredom or other relationship problems, hot flashes causing sleep loss and chronic fatigue, not feeling well in general, and pain with sex in particular. A decline in sexual interest is commonly related to a decline in a partner's sexual desire or sexual capability. These, and other things you've probably already added to my list, put sex way down on your agenda. But for purposes of this discussion, let's just say that sexual interest is indeed present. Cut me some slack here so we can talk about response instead of no sex at all.

The dominant sexual response researchers of our time have been Dr. Virginia Masters and Dr. William Johnson. Their work done more than 25 years ago is still quite valid and accepted. You may recall their description of the female sexual response stages as excitement, plateau, orgasm, and resolution.

✦ During *sexual excitement* in women, pelvic blood vessels dilate which congests the area with blood. This results in vaginal lubrication, as secretions pour out through the walls of your vagina. Muscles begin to tense. This is the "Mm hmm" stage.

✦ In the *plateau* phase, arousal increases dramatically, causing a rapid heart rate, swelling of the clitoris from blood engorgement, dilation and lengthening in the upper vagina, and tensing of the muscles surrounding the lower vagina. This is the "For god's sake don't stop!" phase.

✦ *Orgasm* is the peak moment of sexual response. Rhythmic contractions of the uterus and lower vagina occur, and enjoyment may be exquisite. There may be multiple peaks or a single high. Intensity varies all the way from "That was nice" to "That was showtime."

✦ In *resolution*, pelvic vascular congestion quickly subsides if orgasm has occurred, and a feeling of relaxation washes over you. Peace and warmth and closeness are maximal. If orgasm did not happen, resolution takes longer. During this time, hypersensitivity may occur in the genital structures, particularly the clitoris. This is usually brief or nonexistent, and repeat arousal with additional orgasms is possible.

The above pattern of sexual response remains unchanged throughout life, although the individual components may vary with the passage of time. Lubrication may have taken only seconds at age 20, whereas it could be 5–15 minutes 20 to 30 years later. Some women who complain of vaginal dryness may only be suffering from not enough foreplay, although estrogen deficiency is also a well-proven cause. Orgasms may not be as intense or as reliable. The number of orgasmic contractions may be diminished from two or three, to one or two. Clitoral sensitivity may be lessened by diminished blood flow and fewer neurologic connections. So sexual response may be specifically altered after menopause, generally four to five years after the last period. Given enough sexual stimulation, however, women at any age can be responsive. Dr. Ruth Weg, a gerontologist (specialist in aging) at the University of Southern California, sagely remarks, "Genital response is only one measure of the total sexual experience." Caring and sharing and intimacy have major roles to play as well.

CHANGES IN ANATOMY

Anatomic genital changes result from withdrawal of estrogen support. Recall from the discussion in Chapter 8 that your vagina and vulva are dependent on estrogen to maintain normal anatomy and function. Regular sexual stimulation is also a factor. You can confirm this if you recall how sex made your vagina tender after a period of abstinence. After estrogen slowdown, blood supply diminishes and tissue thinning begins. Vaginal changes are characterized by thinning of the lining tissue. Up to 90% of the thickness may be lost. Elasticity is also lost in this process. This results in a narrower and shorter vagina. When advanced vaginal atrophy has occurred, it may not be possible to insert even a finger. The functional effect of these anatomic changes is less vaginal lubrication from sexual stimulation and pain with intercourse. The vaginal acidity (pH), which reduces resistance to bacterial and yeast infections, is raised.

The vulvar folds outside your vagina also may be affected. The outer folds (labia majora) and inner folds (labia minora) become thin and inelastic. Loss of fat under the skin makes the labia smaller and flatter. Your clitoris becomes less sensitive to stimulation because of a decreased blood supply and fewer functioning nerve endings. Vulvar dryness may cause a very itchy condition called *pruritus*; this can be very frustrating.

Attempting to have sex in the presence of vulvar and vaginal atrophy can result in bruising and lacerations because of the friction from dryness and inelasticity. Some women who have had one or more episodes of painful sex will anticipate a recurrence of the pain with such dread that they have severe involuntary vaginal muscle spasms called *vaginismus*, making penetration impossible. All of this sounds awful, I must admit, but it doesn't happen to every woman. It isn't a process that suddenly grabs you without notice. Dr. Lila Nachtigall and Joan Heilman of the New York University Medical Center reported in 1995 that although this process starts at menopause, or before, only 25% of women have vaginal dryness five years later.

Your cervix and uterus become smaller after menopause. Some women report that subsequent orgasmic contractions are painful, but this is not frequent.

Prevention and Treatment

Help for improving the anatomic and physiologic sexual changes of menopause can involve quite a number of modalities:

1. lubricants
2. maintaining regular sexual stimulation about twice per week
3. vaginal dilators
4. Kegel exercises
5. hormone replacement therapy

Excellent lubricants are available without prescription: K-Y jelly, Replens, Astroglide, and saliva (not sold in stores!) are among the best. Petroleum jelly works OK, but it weakens latex condoms and may disguise the early signs of vaginal infection. If you feel ill at ease about using a lubricant, or somehow defeated by the need for one, introduce it as part of sex play. Most partners readily and enthusiastically embrace lubricant use. It may even become part of your sex vocabulary: "Let's go home and get K-Y'd" or "How would you like to Astroglide?" Lubricants can be very helpful in facilitating pleasurable sex, although they have no effect in preventing vaginal atrophy.

Sexual frequency alone can keep your vagina in good functioning condition because the sexual stimulation prevents chronic dryness. If you do not have a partner, self-stimulation will work too, since lubrication is produced and the same muscles contract as in partnered sex. Masters and Johnson recommend one or two sexual episodes per week. They were the ones who coined the phrase "use it or lose it."

A vaginal dilator can prove quite useful in preventing shrinking and shortening. These are penis-shaped forms of varying size, which can be purchased in pharmacies and surgical supply stores. They have been used extensively after irradiation for cancer to prevent vaginal shrinking. A vibrator can serve the same purpose. They work best if used about three times per week, combined with self-stimulation or a pelvic muscle squeezing routine called Kegel exercises (see below). If you have gone several months without vaginal sex, the dilator can be useful before resumption of sex. Better, though, to have used it all during the time of the abstinence. Better still to make it a regular habit.

Kegel exercises were developed by a urologist, Dr. Arnold Kegel, in the early 1950s. The exercise strengthens the pelvic floor muscles, called *pubococcygeus* (PC), and helps control a type of involuntary urine loss called stress incontinence. It involves squeezing the muscles around your vagina, urethra, and anus. These are the same muscles you must use to cut off urine flow but without squeezing your legs together. As a matter of fact, that's how you teach yourself the exercise. After you know which muscles to use, you do not need to be passing urine to do Kegels. Just squeeze, hold for 5–10 seconds, and relax. Do a set of 10 repetitions, and gradually work up to about 3–5 sets each day. Many sex therapists recommend doing a set of "flutter" Kegel exercises daily. Here you squeeze, squeeze, squeeze as fast as you can. Kegels are helpful in controlling stress incontinence; it turns out that they are also quite beneficial in improving sexual sensitivity and vaginal control. They improve the tone of pelvic muscles. Men are also helped by Kegel exercises in improved erections. Be sure to tell him. The nice thing about this exercise is that you don't have to change into your sneakers and sweats to do it. No one ever knows you are working out.

The most difficult part about Kegels is remembering to do them. Therefore, it is a good idea to use daily events as a reminder: taking a shower, brushing your teeth, waiting for a traffic light, standing in line, when your telephone call is on ignore, etc. Several years ago, one of my patients who had been doing the exercises was in the office. I inquired about her progress and asked if she was remembering to do them. She told me her job involved meeting the public quite a bit, and her routine was to dash off a set of Kegel exercises whenever an attractive man happened on the scene—said it made her job infinitely more interesting.

An alternative to Kegel exercises is the use of vaginal weights. These are a series of five cone-shaped weights, resembling tampons, that are graduated in weight from 20 to 70 grams. You place the smallest in your vagina for ten to fifteen minutes twice daily. The muscles you need to strengthen are the ones needed to prevent the weight from falling out. Starting from a sitting position, you gradually work up to standing. When you can retain the weight even when laughing or coughing, you are ready to progress to the next weight. They are called Femina Pelvic Muscle Training Weights and cost about $100. They can be purchased from Dacomed Corporation in Minneapolis, MN, (800) 328-1103.

Hormone replacement therapy with estrogen, if started in a timely fashion, can prevent most of the problems we have been discussing. Estrogen can also relieve them if they are already established. Estrogen restores vaginal moisture, as well as normal vaginal wall thickness and elasticity. Vulvar skin dryness clears up. Painful sex will disappear in about a month if atrophy is not too far advanced. With a normal vaginal pH, fewer infections occur.

Testosterone, the male hormone, is increasingly being used to improve sexual desire. It is now known that testosterone is the engine of sexual motivation, sexual desire, and sexual fantasies in *both genders*. Estrogen's role is more involved with sexual responses such as arousal, lubrication, and orgasm. If you are well estrogenized, meaning no vaginal dryness or thinning, yet your sexual desire has plummeted, a trial of testosterone is well worth it. If you use testosterone supplements, you will generally experience improved sexual desire and increased fantasies. In addition, depression is lessened, memory is improved, moods are elevated, and your energy level is higher (Ploutte 1994). Should testosterone fail to improve these parameters, other causes should be strongly considered. These include hypothyroidism, an overproduction of a pituitary hormone called prolactin, or psychiatric disorders such as depression and anxiety. Marital and situational problems may also be the source.

If you feel uneasy about initiating a trial of testosterone, a blood test to measure free testosterone will give a good clue. Your testosterone level needs to be in the range of 30–60 nanograms/ml to sustain optimal sexual desire. If it is below 30, treatment with 1–2 mg of testosterone taken 3–6 times per week can make a big difference. The tablet form can lower your good guy high-density lipoprotein (HDL), but this is caused by higher doses. Pellets placed under the skin can serve the same purpose without lowering the HDL. A skin patch is available but it has been designed for men, and the dose is too high for women. If less than 50–75 mg per month is taken, undesirable side effects can be avoided such as facial hair, deeper voice, acne, weight gain.

Summing Up

Menopause is not the end of the road for sex. A gradual change may begin at this time, but it need not be fatal to good sex. Effective help is available in abundance, for both prevention and treatment. The old cultural perception that midlife women are unattractive, and therefore not sexually desirable, is being blown out of the water. Midlife sexual role models are setting a new standard, so you don't have to accept your previously assigned role any longer. You and your partner, having realized this, will forge new and enduring bonds of intimacy and respect. Then, with your relationship and your sexuality intact, you can proceed with confidence to your great life ahead.

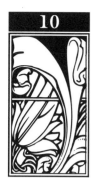

SEX AND MEN
AT MIDLIFE
ALSO CHANGED, BUT ALIVE AND WELL

This chapter's purpose is to acquaint you with the sexuality changes that men undergo. Men are affected emotionally and physically by these time-mediated changes, just as you are. Your being aware of your partner's altered sexuality and what can be done to help will aid in integrating both of you into a relationship that can remain durable and satisfying.

A Crisis of Performance

Time brings change for men too. It is much more gradual than for women but of no less concern. The physical changes eventually make a significant impact on sex with resultant emotional turmoil for him, and perhaps for you as a couple. The words that best characterize the male experience are *diminished prowess*:

- erections take longer to achieve and require more direct penile stimulation
- maintaining an erection is often a problem, which limits the duration of sex. For some men, the opposite is true, with delayed orgasm. This turns out to be great for partners who also require more time
- after ejaculation, erections fade quickly
- resolution and readiness for another erection may require several hours to a day, or more

HE NEEDS HELP TOO

Just as you do, men need reassurance that their changed sexuality is understood and accepted as a new aspect of the relationship. It's OK and natural for time to be transforming him somewhat. Reassurance will be very helpful and necessary in preserving his feeling that he remains sexually attractive to you.

WERE MASTERS AND JOHNSON WRONG?

Abraham Morgentaler thinks so. He is the director of the male infertility and impotence program at Boston's Beth Israel Hospital. In 1996, he stated that Masters and Johnson, in their sexual behavior study carried out in the 1960s, described impotence as a mental rather than physical problem. This fostered the now widely held belief that impotence is a personal, moral, and psychological failure. Morgentaler and others believe that impotence is the result of a body part failing. A cascade of other psychological, interpersonal, and social problems then descends from the failure. If it is a failed body part, there may be remedies for many men.

Prevention and Treatment

Several avenues for improvement regarding "diminished prowess" changes exist.

✦ *Treatment for high blood pressure.* Men who have high blood pressure may experience diminished erection capability as a side effect of antihypertensive medication. A discussion with the prescribing doctor is certainly appropriate.

✦ *Stimulation.* Inadequate erections or delayed erections can be much improved by direct stimulation of the penis, orally or manually. If manual, use of a lubricant will be very pleasurable for him, and mutual use of lubricants will give pleasure to both of you.

✦ *Kegel exercises.* This involves squeezing the same muscles as for stopping urine flow or for expelling the final amounts of urine at the end of urination. As with Kegels for women, it should be the same routine of squeezing for 5–10 seconds, relax and repeat. Over time, a set of 10 contractions around 4–6 times daily may slowly make a difference. He will probably have the same problems remembering to do Kegel exercises as you do, so let daily events be the trigger: shaving, showering, traffic lights (could be interesting if you're both sitting there dashing off a set of Kegels), reading the paper, watching TV, etc. Patience is required because progress is slow, but with persistence, men notice improved sexual sensitivity, better erections, and more control.

✦ *Penile implants.* Permanent impotence may occur in men who have had prostate surgery or vascular bypass operations on pelvic blood vessels. It can also be a consequence of severe hardening of the arteries such as can occur with diabetes. A penile implant, while not trouble-free, may be the answer. These vary all the way from a simple malleable rodlike device to sophisticated hydraulic implants that can produce an erection whenever and for as long as desired. A surgical operation is, of course, needed for this, and that can be expensive. Insurance covers the procedure in certain circumstances. Consult a urologist or a plastic surgeon about it.

✦ *Vacuum devices.* A variety of vacuum devices are being used as alternatives to penile implants. The penis is inserted into a tube, a vacuum is applied causing blood to engorge the penis just as in a natural erection, and a constriction ring is placed at the base of the penis. This prevents blood from leaving the penis and sustains an erection. Manufacturers suggest limiting use of the constriction to about 30 minutes. Satisfying sex has been reported by the majority of users. At $350–$400, vacuum devices are much less expensive than surgical procedures and allow you to avoid an operation. One such device called Response II is marketed by Mentor Urology, Inc., 5425 Hollister Avenue, Santa Barbara, CA 93111, (800) 235–5731. Your doctor can prescribe it, and your pharmacist will supply it. Medicare will cover the cost.

✦ *Injections.* A shot in the penis can help. "A *shot* in the penis?" Yes, you heard right. A drug called *alprostadil* is marketed by Pharmacia & Upjohn under the brand name Caverject. It does a good job in producing adequate erections, which are well sustained for a long enough time to have satisfying sex. Dr. Perry Nadig, a urologist in San Antonio, Texas, found that 86% of men were satisfied with the results. The injection is self-administered each time an erection is desired. Most fair observers would have to admit, however, that interrupting foreplay for your partner to stab his penis with a needle could be a bit distracting.

✦ *Drug therapy.* A pill for impotence is under study by researchers at Pfizer Inc. In preliminary studies, they found over 80% of men reported improvement in quality of erections. The generic name for this drug is *sildenafil.* When marketed in the late '90s, the brand name will be Viagra.

✦ *Hormone replacement.* HRT for men has been considered, but very little research on this has been done in the United States. Most of it to date has been done in Europe where they call it *androtherapy.*

Androgens (male hormones) are generally assessed by measuring blood levels of testosterone. These levels gradually diminish over about 30 years starting in the 40s. By age 60, significant lowering has usually occurred. The normal male testosterone level is between 300 and 1,200 ng/ml., as compared to yours at 80–90. A level below 500 ng/ml in men generally coincides with such changes as altered sexual capability, decreased muscle mass and strength, osteoporotic bone loss, and diminished vitality. Well, the answer would seem to be give those dudes HRT, right? Maybe. Testosterone lowers good guy HDL, and raises bad guy LDL—the opposite effect that estrogen has on women. Testosterone worsens the risk of prostate cancer, a very common tumor in aging men. At this point, there are not enough hard data to know with any assurance how to proceed with HRT in men, but studies are ongoing.

Communication . . . Once Again the Key to Success

Many women who are going through menopause-related changes of their own, misinterpret their partner's problems as lack of interest. This is not usually the case at all. Men have very fragile sexual egos. They tend to be quite embarrassed about their evolving crisis of performance and talk little about it. Now is the time to talk, though. A man needs to be reassured that you understand he also is not in control of whether or not he ages, that love and closeness won't be conditioned on the quality of erections, and that love and closeness may not even be conditioned on intercourse.

Once men and women recognize that sex may change with the passage of years, that sexual response may take more time and attention for both genders, that orgasm intensity and frequency may diminish, that vaginal dryness and erection problems are not the end of the road for sex, *then* a couple can start addressing what they can do to integrate their altered situation into their desire for continued sexuality. That we undergo change and our sexuality is altered is undeniable. It happens to both sexes, although at differing rates of change. We also have gender differences as to what the changes mean to each partner and what they mean to each couple. You worry that vaginal change and the subsequent diminished sexual desire will affect your sexual desirability. Likewise, a man worries that poor erections and poorly sustained erections will adversely affect *his* sexual desirability.

Talking about it can wash away the anxiety of change, by each educating the other about his or her needs, and by each giving the other permission to change. The closeness that results from honest communication can be magic, just like the intimacy of an honest hug—very healing.

Summing Up

So, men change too. The rate of change differs from yours, but it is change nonetheless. Various treatment modalities and techniques for either partner can make a significant difference in improving the changes and in improving sexuality. It is not necessary to let a disturbing situation become hopeless. When you emerge from your midlife transition with your relationship intact, a new sexuality can also blossom that will be satisfying for both of you far into the future.

SECTION III

MANAGEMENT CHOICES

In this section we will get to the actual treatment options and management choices. Hormone replacement therapy, alternative therapies, stress management, and fitness are covered. Hysterectomy, chemotherapy, and premature menopause are also discussed. In Chapter 16, I have made suggestions for selecting the appropriate health care adviser to help you answer your menopausal questions and clarify your management options. Chapter 17, which discusses midlife changes for men and men's involvement in their partner's midlife changes, is a chapter that I encourage men to read. The final chapter is about the other side of your menopausal transition—the good news about the great life ahead.

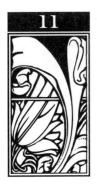

HORMONE REPLACEMENT THERAPY (HRT)
TO USE, OR NOT TO USE

Hormone replacement therapy is the cornerstone of postmenopausal management. HRT has fervent supporters and passionate detractors, and each camp
has its own reasons for its stance. This chapter will give you a look at both the
benefits and the drawbacks of hormone use, plus a listing of the indications
and contraindications. You will learn the several types of regimens and
hormone combinations. Generic and brand names are used, as are the commonly prescribed dosages. The science supporting, and failing to support,
HRT is cited.

HRT—An Overview

NOT ENOUGH WOMEN USE HRT

A study by Dr. D. T. Felson and coworkers in 1993 showed that the
continuation rate in taking hormone replacement therapy is a major problem.
National statistics indicate that 60% of women who start HRT will stop within
a year. Somewhere around 20%–30% never get their prescriptions filled. Of
those who do take hormones, 90% will have stopped using them by the end
of seven years. Why such a sorry record for HRT? On the part of menopausal
women, fear of cancer and irregular bleeding are the most frequently cited
reasons. My personal opinion is that in addition to these reasons, and perhaps
aggravating them, women have been poorly educated about menopause in

general and about HRT in particular. That is a sad commentary on the health care givers who provide services and on our obligation to educate. We have not effectively countered misinformation nor dispelled cultural myths and public skepticism. So, I urge you to inform yourself in every way possible about menopause and how to manage your transition through it. You will make much better decisions if you are informed. You will then be much more comfortable with whatever course you set for yourself.

HRT GIVES YOU AN EDGE

To help you decide about HRT, the advantages and disadvantages will be considered as well as the contraindications. The following list of advantages is not merely a consensus of opinion, it is a representation of the scientific study that generated them. The advantages of HRT are

+ improved lipid profile of HDL, LDL, and total cholesterol. There is protection (but not immunity) against cardiovascular disease such as heart attack, stroke, hardening of the arteries, and high blood pressure
+ prevention of osteoporosis and the risk of fractures
+ relief from thinning of vagina, vulva, bladder, and urethra
+ relief from hot flashes
+ improved sleep, short-term memory, sexuality, and sense of well-being
+ reduction in skin aging (not prevention, not reversal)
+ increase in longevity via decreased frequency of potentially fatal problems such as heart attack, stroke, osteoporosis, endometrial cancer
+ reduction of the adverse response to stress. This benefit is reduced slightly when estrogen is combined with a progestin, but only slightly (Lindheim 1994)
+ improvement of memory in postmenopausal women (Robinson 1994)
+ possible reduction in the risk of Alzheimer's disease (Paganinni-Hill & Henderson 1994)

The last three benefits listed above are associated with improved brain function. The studies cited were small, and their results must be regarded as suggestive rather than nailed-to-the-wall, solid evidence. No one is claiming that estrogen replacement will make rocket scientists out of postmenopausal women who are not already rocket scientists. But if it improves brain function or prevents brain deterioration, that's a winner.

Does all that sound good? You bet. The benefit of estrogen in your body is so dramatic, and the loss of it is so threatening, that HRT seems to far outweigh any other method as the primary route of menopausal management. My opinion is that you and every woman should understand the HRT option and should be *offered* HRT unless there are specific health problems contra-indicating it. The ball is in your court as to whether it is, or is not, right for you.

BUT HRT CAN BE RISKY TOO

As for drawbacks to estrogen use in HRT, a 1992 technical bulletin of the American College of Obstetricians and Gynecologists (ACOG) listed a number of significant conditions that can result in a recommendation that you not use this option.

Abnormal vaginal bleeding

HRT is contraindicated in the case of abnormal vaginal bleeding that suggests a disease process. This abnormality should be investigated with a biopsy of the uterine lining and resolved before you begin HRT. A D&C (scraping of the uterine lining) could also be necessary if the biopsy is abnormal. Both of these procedures can be done in an office setting through a hysteroscope, a lighted tube placed in your cervix through which can be seen the inside of your uterus. If you should be unlucky enough to have abnormal bleeding from an en-dometrial cancer, taking estrogen could worsen it. Sometimes, taking estrogen in the presence of a previously unknown uterine cancer will make it bleed. This leads to an earlier investigation and diagnosis, with an improved chance for a cure.

Estrogen dependent tumors

Some breast, ovarian, and endometrial cancers have profuse estrogen recep-tors. Taking estrogen can enhance their growth. This is not true for cancer of the cervix or precancerous lesions of the cervix. Uterine fibroids are benign (noncancerous) tumors in the wall of the uterus that may grow with a high dose HRT regimen. Fibroids tend not to grow with the contemporary low dose regimens, to be described later in the chapter.

Liver dysfunction

Impaired liver function from either ongoing hepatitis or damage to the liver from prior disease can make HRT troublesome. Estrogen taken orally passes through the liver after it is absorbed from the intestinal tract, and this may stress an already overtaxed organ. In this situation, the estrogen skin patch would be a better choice, since this route of administration bypasses the liver. Another route that avoids the intestinal tract, and therefore bypasses the liver, is the use of pellets implanted under the skin. This method is being used in Europe but is not yet available in the United States. Although it would conveniently bypass the liver, intramuscular injection of estrogen is rarely used on a regular basis because of the inconvenience, expense, and wide fluctuations in hormone blood levels from one shot to the next.

Previous thromboembolism

This is a blood clot that has lodged in the lung or brain, or a condition that predisposes you to thromboembolism such as phlebitis or certain abnormal heart rhythms. If you have had thrombophlebitis in the distant past from a nonrecurring cause such as injury, or surgery, it is OK to take HRT.

SOME MYTHS AND CONFUSIONS DISPELLED

A few other health conditions that may be ongoing at the same time that HRT is being considered should be discussed. The following are situations where confusion and disagreement as to whether HRT should be offered or withheld have existed (Speroff 1994).

Established coronary heart disease

Low dose estrogen, as currently prescribed for HRT, has a proven beneficial effect on many of the very things that cause coronary disease. These are improved lipid profile, dilation of blood vessels, inhibition of cholesterol deposits on the artery walls, protection against blood clots, improved contracting ability of heart muscle, and improved glucose metabolism. With improved glucose metabolism, the levels of circulating insulin decrease. Insulin causes cholesterol deposits in arteries. So estrogen can prevent worsening of coronary disease; however, it does not reverse an existing condition. The American Heart Association and cardiologists have been reluctant to advise estrogen/progestin use for women who have coronary heart disease. Their position is now changing, since the beneficial effects of HRT have been shown to be related to the low dosages used. Dr. Dean Ornish, a well-known cardiologist at the University of California at San Francisco, has a program for reversal of coronary disease (Ornish 1990). His regimen does not exclude HRT use, although successful reversal of CVD is not attributed to the estrogen.

High blood cholesterol

Estrogen lowers total cholesterol, raises HDL (the good guy) and lowers LDL (the bad guy). The addition of progestin slightly decreases the beneficial effect of the raised HDL, but not much. There is no adverse effect on LDL from adding progestin. If you have a high triglyceride level (a special risk factor for CVD in women), oral estrogen may raise it further, but the estrogen skin patch avoids this. Oral androgens (male hormone) lower triglycerides quite well but they also lower HDL, so androgen must be used with some caution and in tiny doses. Nonoral androgens do not have this negative effect on HDL.

Women with unfavorable lipid profiles also benefit from a low-fat diet and exercise. Some may require cholesterol-lowering drugs.

Diabetes

Estrogen improves glucose metabolism and thereby decreases the amount of time that insulin must circulate in your bloodstream to regulate blood sugar. That's good for our team, so don't let anybody talk you out of it if you are diabetic and menopausal and want hormone replacement. Diabetics do better using transdermal (skin patch) estrogen, because they have a higher than average risk of gall bladder disease, which oral estrogen can enhance.

High blood pressure

Oral estrogen lowers blood pressure slightly by causing the smooth muscle in the blood vessel wall to relax. It facilitates this effect by helping to modulate the release of nitric oxide (a dilator) and endothelin (a constrictor). With the vessels relaxed, the resistance to the flow of blood is reduced because it takes less pressure to force blood through them. Estrogen should not be regarded as a substitute for your blood pressure medication. However, it is not justified to withhold estrogen from you if wish to take it. One note of caution is that about 5% of women who take oral conjugated estrogens (Premarin) will have a rise in blood pressure. This is transient and reversible by discontinuing it. In this situation, the oral route must not be used. The transdermal patch will not cause this effect, so it is not necessary to abandon HRT.

Osteoporosis

In women who already have significant bone loss, especially more than 30%, estrogen is still quite useful. Conjugated estrogen (Premarin) is the best documented oral estrogen, but others can be used (see below). Estrogen plus calcium should ideally be taken for the long term because when they are stopped, rapid bone loss promptly resumes. If you were already behind in bone mass when you began HRT, you will soon be in jeopardy for fractures when you quit.

Gall bladder disease

Estrogen increases this risk, just as was the case when you were on birth control pills. Estrogen increases the amount of cholesterol in the bile produced by your liver, and this promotes the formation of cholesterol gall stones. The estrogen dosage in HRT is about 75% lower than the low dose birth control pill, so you are safer in using it. The skin patch is a better route for women at higher risk for gall bladder disease because the liver is bypassed when the estrogen is initially absorbed into your bloodstream.

Blood clots

The bad rap on estrogen and blood clots came in the 1960s when high dose birth control pills were in use. They did indeed encourage blood clots, which caused strokes and heart attacks. The newer generation of low dose birth control pills does not cause such a risk. They have been approved by the FDA for you to use up to age 50, if you are healthy and a nonsmoker. The estrogen dosage in HRT is far less than even these latest low dose oral contraceptives. So, are they safe? Yes. Nevertheless, if you have had thrombophlebitis in the past, caution is still necessary when considering HRT. The patch would be the preferable route to take estrogen. You can also use estrogen vaginal cream or the estrogen vaginal ring, but this provides hormone replacement for only the vagina and urinary tract.

Varicose veins

Estrogen does not cause varicose veins—period. It does not make you more susceptible to them, and it does not make them worse if you already have them. HRT is safe because the low dose of estrogen used does not increase the risk of blood clots in these veins.

Endometriosis

This is a chronic condition that is very painful. It occurs when uterine lining tissue has located itself outside the uterus on structures such as the fallopian tubes, ovaries, pelvic lining tissue, and intestines. Pain is caused by bleeding and the scarring that results from this abnormally located tissue. Endometriosis is very estrogen sensitive, so it becomes inactive after menopause. Will it recur with HRT? About 5% of women with previous endometriosis will have a recurrence, so careful monitoring is advisable. Some do best on a smaller-than-usual dose that will control menopausal symptoms yet not reactivate the endometriosis.

Cataracts

A University of Wisconsin study found that cataracts were reduced by 10% in women who had taken estrogen for at least five years and by 35% for those who had taken it for 20 years. Cataract prevention also is enhanced by a diet high in antioxidants such as vitamin E, vitamin C, and beta-carotenes.

Arthritis

Women taking HRT have a 30% lower risk of developing arthritis. Even in those who do get arthritis, the severity is much less. Many women who have established arthritis have dramatically improved symptoms after starting estrogen.

Alzheimer's disease

A University of Southern California study of nearly 9,000 postmenopausal women recently found that those treated with estrogen were 40% less likely to develop this disease. And when Alzheimer's did occur, it was of a milder degree in women who were estrogen users.

Estrogen and stress

In 1992, a study by Lindheim, Legro, and Bernstein reported in the *American Journal of Obstetrics & Gynecology* that estrogen reduced the adverse response to stress in postmenopausal women. It is known that stress causes the release of adrenaline and catecholamines, the chemicals that mediate the stress responses in your body. Over time, they harm your heart and blood vessels. Postmenopausal women have a greater reactivity to stress than premenopausal women, and estrogen dampens this. More information is needed to confirm this, but it seems to be yet another cardiovascular protective mechanism of estrogen.

Types of Estrogen

HUMAN ESTROGENS

Your body makes three different estrogens:

✦ *17-beta estradiol* is the major biologically active estrogen made by your ovaries. It has its effect at receptor sites on trillions of cells throughout your body. This is the hormone that declines during perimenopause and is 80%–90% lost by the time of menopause. Pure 17-beta estradiol is now commercially available in a tablet called Estrace and in the skin patches Estraderm, Climara, and Vivelle.

✦ *Estrone* is a weak strogen produced by your ovaries from precursors made in your adrenal glands. This is the form of estrogen made from conversion of precursors in fat cells. Estrone is weaker than estradiol but still biologically active. Estrone can be converted to estradiol by your liver, so in that sense this hormone serves as a reservoir for estradiol. After menopause, estrone continues to be available from fat conversion, which explains why obese women have less osteoporosis and also why they are more at risk for endometrial cancer. It is commercially available in tablets as Ogen and Ortho-Est.

✦ *Estriol* is the weakest estrogen. It is produced in large amounts during pregnancy but otherwise does not circulate in measurable amounts.

Estriol has not been FDA approved for hormone replacement because of inadequate effectiveness.

ANIMAL ESTROGENS

Pregnant mare's urine is loaded with estrogens, just as in pregnant women, and is the source of conjugated equine estrogens marketed as Premarin. Conjugated estrogens actually comprise a group of ten or more. Some of them are close enough to human estrogen that they are useful and effective for hormone replacement. Conjugated estrogens are not as uniform in their effect on various cells as estradiol is. For example, they may work well in restoring vaginal moisture, while at the same time not well enough to adequately improve moodiness. An adverse side effect of equine conjugated estrogens may last longer than with estradiol because they stay in your body for 12 to 14 weeks after the last dose. Estradiol declines after one day. Recent studies have shown that equine estrogens may be more potent than estradiol in raising friendly HDL and lowering unfriendly LDL. There has also been some interest in some properties of equine estrogens that resemble the anti–breast cancer qualities of Tamoxifen, the drug used for prevention of breast cancer recurrence. Conjugated estrogens have now been synthesized but not yet marketed in the United States. Premarin has a good record of effectiveness in HRT, which is why it is in such widespread use.

PLANT ESTROGENS

These are called *phytoestrogens*. Over 300 plants contain phytoestrogens, which are actually precursor molecules from which your body can create estrogen. Soy beans are the most potent food source, while ginseng and dong quai are frequently used herbs with estrogenic activity. See Chapter 12 for a more detailed discussion of these herbs. The potency of estrogenic effect from plants is sufficient to relieve symptoms of estrogen decline in many women, but they do not protect sufficiently against CVD or osteoporosis. Japanese women consume high quantities of soy products in their diet and have far fewer symptoms of estrogen deficiency.

SYNTHETIC ESTROGENS

A lot of confusion exists about the word "synthetic." Many loud voices proclaim that anything made in a laboratory is not "natural" and therefore should be shunned. Nevertheless, it is possible for a laboratory to make estradiol that is precisely the same as your own native ovarian hormone. Estrace is such a product. That makes it "natural," except perhaps for those whose agenda is pure and simple anticommercial anything. There are two synthetic estrogens that are not natural because they do not chemically resemble human estradiol:

+ *Ethinyl estradiol* does not chemically resemble human estradiol and is much more potent than your native hormone. It is most commonly used in birth control pills. This product is stronger than is necessary for HRT and therefore is little used in our country for it. It is commercially available as Estinyl.
+ *Estradiol valerate* is about 100 times more potent than human estradiol, so it is rarely used for HRT in the United States. This is the estrogen used in the Swedish study that reported higher breast cancer rates.

Table 11-1 lists the commonly used estrogens available on the market.

DESIGNER ESTROGENS

Research is currently in an advanced stage on a new type of estrogen designed to avoid the receptor sites in breast and uterine tissue. It will specifically target bone receptor sites (Brody 1997). Several such drugs are in the pipeline now, but one, called *raloxifene*, is in final clinical trials prior to marketing. This is an astonishing breakthrough in estrogen replacement therapy and one that has the potential to allay the concerns women have had about breast and uterine cancer while still offering osteoporosis protection.

Table 11-1
COMMERCIALLY AVAILABLE ESTROGEN PREPARATIONS

Brand name	Type of estrogen	Method of use and dosage
Premarin	Conjugated equine estrogen 45% estrone sulfate, 55% equine estrogens	*Oral tablet:* 0.3, 0.625, 0.9, 1.25, 2.5 mg *Vaginal cream:* 1 g = 0.625 mg
Estrace	Micronized estradiol	*Oral tab.:* 0.5, 1.0, 2.0 mg *Vag. cream:* 1 g = 0.2 mg
Ogen (same as Ortho-Est)	Estropipate (estrone sulfate combined with piperazine)	*Oral tab.:* 0.75, 1.25, 3.0 mg *Vag. cream:* 1 g = 1.5 mg
Estratab (similar to Menest)	Esterified estrogens 85% estrone, 15% equine estrogens	*Oral tab.:* 0.625, 1.25, 2.5 mg *Vag. cream:* 1 g = 0.625 mg
Estraderm	Estradiol	*Skin patch:* 0.05, 0.1 mg
Climara	Estradiol	*Skin patch:* 0.05, 0.1 mg
Vivelle	Estradiol	*Skin patch:* 0.0375, 0.05, 0.075, 0.1 mg

Estrogen Routes

ORAL ESTROGEN

This is far and away the most common method. Premarin has been available since 1941, and since it has been the most widely used, it has also been the most widely studied. The 0.625 mg Premarin tablet is the most frequently prescribed for HRT because it is the minimum dose that prevents osteoporosis. Plant estrogens have been used to derive the estradiol used in Estrace and Estraderm (skin patch). The laboratory produced estradiol is the same as your native ovarian estradiol. Synthetic and semisynthetic compounds have been used in Ogen, Ortho-Est, and Estratab. Any of these may be legitimately prescribed by your doctor.

TRANSDERMAL ESTROGEN

Estrogen replacement via an adhesive skin patch has been a marvelous option for women who must not take estrogen orally. It allows estrogen to bypass the liver and be absorbed through the skin directly into the bloodstream. When estrogen does not pass through the intestinal tract and the liver, it cannot cause the release of liver enzymes which may aggravate preexisting high blood pressure. This route also avoids the risk of thrombophlebitis and gall bladder disease. Transdermal estrogen maintains a steadier blood level of estradiol because of slow constant release from the patch. Research shows that the patch is just as effective as oral estrogen as long as your skin absorbs enough hormone.

Estraderm, the most commonly used patch, must be changed twice weekly and is best tolerated by your skin when applied to the abdomen, buttocks, or thigh. You can control skin irritation by allowing the alcohol in the patch to dry briefly before applying it or by changing the location of the patch. If it comes off in the shower or while swimming, just reapply it. The water will not alter its effectiveness. The patch contains estradiol, which is the native estrogen produced by your ovaries.

Two newer patches called Climara and Vivelle are now available. These patches are smaller, thinner, more transparent, adhere better, and are more flexible than Estraderm. They need replacement only once weekly. The lower dose Climara and Vivelle patches do not deliver enough estradiol to maintain your blood level over 50 pg/ml, which is the minimum needed to prevent osteoporosis. The higher dosages of these patches work quite well however.

About 15%–20% of patch users are troubled with skin irritation. Another problem with the patch is that the amount of estradiol absorbed into your bloodstream can vary by as much as 20% from woman to woman. This is because of differences in skin thickness and penetrability. A lower dose of estrogen may also result if you live in a hot climate where profuse perspiration may wash away the hormone before it enters your skin. Sweating may also present problems with the patch sticking to your skin. In the early stages of patch use, your blood level of estradiol should be monitored to make sure you are getting an adequate dose.

VAGINAL CREAM

Estrogen cream is inserted into your vagina with a measured vaginal applicator. The primary effect of the vaginal route is to improve the symptoms of vaginal and bladder atrophy. The usual dose is one gram of cream twice weekly. At this dose and frequency, however, the vaginal route cannot be counted on to relieve menopausal symptoms or to prevent osteoporosis and CVD. In larger and more frequent doses, estrogen enters your bloodstream in measurable amounts, usually about one-quarter to one-half the equivalent dose taken orally. The vaginal route is being explored as a possible primary method of using HRT. When estrogen is placed in a saline solution and used like a douching preparation, the blood levels achieved are four times higher than with the cream.

VAGINAL RING

Estrogen in a vaginal ring is inserted much like a diaphragm, from which very tiny doses are slowly released. It improves vaginal and bladder symptoms. Very little gets into the general circulation, so perimenopausal symptoms are little changed. This is a Swedish device that was designed for use in women who have had breast cancer. The FDA approved a device called Estring in February 1997 for use in the United States. Work is in progress on a vaginal ring combining both estrogen and progesterone for continuous release HRT.

INJECTIONS

Intramuscular injection of estrogen is rarely used as a long-term method of administration because it is both inconvenient and expensive. In addition, injections are the least reliable method of maintaining a steady level of estrogen in your bloodstream. You go from a very low level at the time of injection to a high level, which then dwindles to a low level again. The most common circumstance for use of injection is immediately after surgery when both ovaries have been removed.

IMPLANTS

Estrogen pellets implanted under the skin have been used in Europe for many years. They last about six months. This practice has not yet been approved by the FDA for use in the United States. With pellet use, it is still necessary to use progesterone to protect your uterus.

TOPICAL GELS

Estrogen in a gel form is still another method widely used in Europe, but it is not yet FDA approved. This is a measured dose of estrogen rubbed into the skin once each day. Once the gel has entered the skin it releases a steady dose of estrogen. This method has been quite popular with European women.

EQUIVALENT ESTROGEN DOSES

Oral conjugated estrogen (Premarin) has been the gold standard for the necessary dose of estrogen in HRT for several decades. The dosages used in the United States are now about half of what they were 20 years ago. In Europe, the standard dose is still double the U.S. dose. Table 11-2 shows the current equivalents of 0.625 mg of conjugated estrogen, which is the dose that works for most women.

Most experts in the field feel that you should be started on the "standard" dose of estrogen and then move up if your hot flashes and other symptoms are not controlled in a reasonable time (four to six weeks). Later you should get back to the standard dose. The adequacy of your dose can be determined by measuring your blood level of estradiol. About 80–100 pg/ml is the desirable level, but the minimum for osteoporosis protection is above 50 pg/ml. The term *standard* refers to the minimum dose that has been shown to prevent osteoporosis, meaning 0.625 mg of conjugated estrogen or an equivalent. This dose is also effective in reducing heart disease.

Table 11-2	
ESTROGEN EQUIVALENTS	
Premarin	0.625 mg
Estrace	1 mg
Estratabs	0.625 mg
Ogen	0.625 mg
Ortho-Est	0.625 mg
Estraderm	0.05 mg
Climara	0.05 mg
Vivelle	0.05 mg

Progesterone

PROGESTERONE AND PROGESTIN . . . WHAT'S THE DIFFERENCE?

Progesterone has been used primarily in a synthetic form called *progestin*, because *natural progesterone* is essentially inactivated in the intestinal tract. Natural progesterone, made from soy beans and wild Mexican yams, has now been micronized (broken down into fine particles) to combat this undesired effect. Natural progesterone was found effective in the Postmenopausal Estrogen/Progestin Interventions (PEPI) Trial reported in 1995. This study of 875 postmenopausal women was conducted in seven medical centers. PEPI studied the use of unopposed estrogen, as well as various combinations of estrogen and progestin. Also looked at was estrogen combined with micronized natural progesterone. The purpose was to determine what effect these hormones would have on cardiovascular disease (CVD) risk factors. The data showed that combined estrogen-progesterone HRT definitely benefits women and reduces the CVD risk that faces every postmenopausal woman. Natural progesterone was slightly more beneficial than the synthetic progestins, but the numbers did not reach statistical significance. PEPI also addressed whether the addition of progestins or natural progesterone would significantly diminish the known estrogen protection. It did, but only slightly, and definitely not to the degree that would make it imprudent to advocate its use. Prevention of uterine cancer is the main advantage of using progestin. This outweighs the disadvantages so dramatically that it leaves unopposed estrogen and "just doing nothing" in the dust.

DRAWBACKS OF PROGESTIN USE

It bears repeating that the major reason for using progestin in HRT is to reduce the risk of endometrial cancer. The data have shown conclusively that it does just that; however, progestin use has well-known disagreeable side effects:

- ◆ sore breasts
- ◆ weight gain
- ◆ irritability
- ◆ fluid retention
- ◆ decreased sexual desire
- ◆ minor depression
- ◆ bloating
- ◆ constipation

These side effects do not happen to everyone, of course, but it is no fun for those who have any of them. They are lessened with micronized natural progesterone. This form of progesterone could be given a trial, if synthetic progestins have any of these effects on you.

Table 11-3		
COMMERCIALLY AVAILABLE PROGESTERONE PREPARATIONS		
Brand name	**Generic name**	**Dosages**
Provera, Cycrin	Medroxyprogesterone acetate (MPA)	2.5, 5.0, 10.0 mg
Aygestin	Norethindrone acetate	5 mg
Micronor	Norethindrone	0.35 mg
Ovrette	Norgestrel	0.075 mg
Natural micronized progesterone	Progesterone	25, 50, 100, 200 mg

Types of Progesterone

Table 11-3 lists the commercially available progesterone preparations.

NATURAL PROGESTERONE

Natural progesterone is considerably more expensive than are progestins and not as readily available. Many physicians have little experience with it as yet, since it is a relatively new product. Micronized progesterone is rapidly metabolized, so it must be taken twice daily to maintain proper blood levels. The usual dose is 200–300 mg per day. Dr. J. T. Hargrove's 1989 study suggested that since it can produce drowsiness, the morning dose should be 100 mg and the evening dose, 200 mg. Both doses should be taken with food. Dose regulation with natural progesterone is much more of a problem than with synthetic progestins. Natural progesterone is not commercially available in the United States, but you can get it from specialty pharmacies. They buy their bulk stock from foreign pharmaceutical companies and make up tablets, creams, and suppositories themselves. One such pharmacy is the

Women's International Pharmacy
5708 Monona Drive
Madison, WI 53716-3152
(800) 279-5708 or (608) 221-7800

PROGESTINS

Provera, one form of *medroxyprogesterone acetate* (MPA), is derived from progesterone and is the most commonly used synthetic version. MPA is also available as Cycrin. Dosages will be discussed below. The most frequent complaint by women who take MPA is the mood swings it can cause, ranging from irritability to depression, so the lowest effective dose should be used.

MPA is available in a variety of tablet doses, so it can be used in either the cyclic or continuous regimens to be discussed below.

Aygestin is derived from testosterone by chemically changing the molecule. It has no malelike effects on women. It is only made in a 5 mg scored tablet, which is equivalent to 10 mg of MPA. The effects and potential side effects are about the same as Provera.

Micronor (*norethindrone*) and Ovrette (*norgestrel*) are both "mini-pills" used primarily as estrogen-free birth control pills. They can be combined with estrogen and used in a continuous regimen wherein you take both hormones every day. There are fewer mood swings with these, but they can lower HDL, so low doses must be used and lipids monitored initially. These are very low dose progestins, and there is concern that they may not be potent enough to protect your endometrium from the thickening that results from hyperplasia. If you use these in HRT, your endometrial thickness should be monitored annually with ultrasound.

Megace (*megestrol acetate*) is a very potent progestin that has primarily been used for treatment of recurrent endometrial and breast cancer. It can relieve hot flashes for those women taking Tamoxifen following breast cancer treatment. Megace has a positive influence on bone density, but in long-term use it may negatively influence lipids. This is a special-use drug which is not regularly employed for HRT.

OTHER FORMS OF PROGESTERONE

The *Progestasert IUD* (intrauterine device) is another method of progesterone use. It delivers a steady daily dose of natural progesterone directly to the uterine lining. The amounts delivered are quite small but still sufficient for protection of the endometrium. Because of the tiny doses delivered, no side effects occur. Similar results were found in another small study reported by Raudaskoski and others in the *American Journal of Obstetrics and Gynecology* in 1995. They used an IUD that is not currently available in the United States. Work on this form of therapy is still preliminary. The drawback is that this IUD only lasts one year and then must be replaced. A Finnish IUD using levonorgestrel lasts seven years, and hopefully will be available in the United States in the near future. IUD insertion is painful, but this can be largely prevented with a local anesthetic.

Progesterone creams have been tried by some women who still have menstrual periods to counter the high estrogen levels in the second half of the cycle. Accurate dosage delivery is problematical with this method, so creams should not be used in postmenopausal HRT as yet. The natural progesterone craze has really taken off in creams. Since natural progesterone is a plant derivative, it is not regulated by the FDA. Currently there are more than two dozen products being marketed with varying amounts of progesterone in them. Many are being hawked as the only treatment necessary for control of postmenopausal osteoporosis. This is an exaggeration of the facts. None of them has been studied in placebo controlled trials, so at this point they do not deserve your patronage or your money.

HRT Regimens

Several administration methods are used for hormone replacement. Most can be grouped under the general headings of

- ✦ unopposed estrogen, where no progestin is used
- ✦ cyclic HRT using both estrogen and progestin in a monthly cycle
- ✦ continuous HRT using both hormones every day

UNOPPOSED ESTROGEN

This regimen was used for several decades until studies in the 1970s demonstrated the connection between estrogen and endometrial cancer of the uterus. That frightened everybody, patient and physician alike. The news media loved it. The usual regimen was Premarin 0.625 mg or 1.25 mg daily, on for three weeks and off for one week. Since then, "estrogen only" has been in the dog house, and very few physicians prescribe it this way. If this regimen *is* used, it is necessary to monitor your endometrium on an annual basis with a vaginal ultrasound scan to measure its thickness. This is a painless office procedure in which a specially designed probe is inserted into your vagina. The thickness of your endometrium is easily and accurately measured, and your ovaries can be assessed at the same time. If your endometrium is less than 5 mm in depth, that's it until next year. If the endometrial depth is over 5 mm, an endometrial biopsy (office procedure) needs to be done (Parsons 1993). Endometrial cancer takes several years to develop, and it will almost always be preceded by hyperplasia, a noncancerous or precancerous thickening. If this is seen on the biopsy tissue, it can be reversed by taking cyclic progestin for a few months. This produces menstrual periods and shedding of the abnormal tissue. A follow-up biopsy is needed to prove the hyperplasia has been replaced with normal tissue.

What most women liked about unopposed estrogen was that they did not have vaginal bleeding, their hot flashes were controlled, and they generally felt great—although the symptoms recurred during the one week in four off estrogen. What they did *not* like were the endometrial biopsies; they hurt. Some preliminary work has been done on using unopposed estrogen, with the addition of progestin (Provera, 10 mg) for two weeks every three months to produce shedding of the endometrium. This could turn out to be a reasonable compromise for women who suffer progestin side effects with combined estrogen-progestin HRT. In 1995, Grady reported that as little as six months use of unopposed estrogen can increase your risk for endometrial cancer fourfold. In addition, the increased risk lingers for several years. If progestin is subsequently added, the risk is reduced but is still about double the normal risk seen in nonhormone users. If estrogen and progestin are combined at the outset of HRT, the risk is the same as in nonhormone users.

CYCLIC HRT

The classic sequential method is to take estrogen (Premarin, 0.625 mg, or Estrace, 1.0 mg) from the first through the 25th day of each month and to add progestin (Provera, 10 mg) to the estrogen for the last 12 of the 25 days. About 80% of women on this method will have withdrawal bleeding late in the month. For women who have progestin side effects (weight gain, sore breasts, fluid retention, mood swings, etc.), the Provera can be lowered to 5 mg. This helps a lot. Most physicians are prescribing 5 mg of Provera now because it offers nearly the same endometrial protection as 10 mg. For women who have progestin side effects even on the lower Provera dose, a progestin-only mini-pill (Micronor), containing 0.35 mg of norethindrone, works quite well. Micronized natural progesterone can possibly serve the same ends.

For women who have hot flashes and other symptoms during the few days when they are off all hormones, another semicyclic regimen can be used. This involves taking estrogen every day and adding progestin for 14 days each month. A new estrogen-progestin regimen called Premphase has been developed for this purpose. It provides a 14-day punch-out card of Premarin plus a second card with a 14-day supply of a tablet containing both Premarin, 0.625 mg, and medroxyprogesterone acetate 5 mg (same as Provera 5 mg). Withdrawal bleeding occurs with this regimen also. For cyclic therapy, this is the one I advocate.

The minimum dose of conjugated estrogen (Premarin) necessary to prevent osteoporosis is generally regarded to be 0.625 mg. A study in the late 1980s reported that 0.3 mg of Premarin, if combined with 1,500 mg of calcium, could prevent osteoporosis; but cyclic progestin was also needed (Ettinger 1987). I still recommend 0.625 mg.

The biggest hurdle I encountered in the early years of using the cyclic regimen was with my patients whose menopause had been many years ago. Now, they were suddenly considering HRT because we had been discussing osteoporosis and heart disease. Inevitably the conversation got to: "Are you crazy, sonny? You want me to start my *periods* again?" I stammered: "Uh, yes ma'am. I guess I do." Felt like a darn fool. There weren't a lot of takers in the late postmenopausal set.

CONTINUOUS HRT

Continuous hormone therapy got me off the hook with elderly post-menopausal women because the majority end up having no monthly bleeding. With this method, both hormones are used every day, 365 days per year. Premarin 0.625 mg, plus Provera 2.5 mg are prescribed. In November 1995, the FDA approved a tablet combining both estrogen and progestin. This will make it much more convenient for the 4.6 million women using the continuous regimen. The combination tablet was marketed as Prempro. Light vaginal bleeding still occurs from time to time for about 50%, but it diminishes and stops altogether after about six months. By the end of a year, 10%–20% of women still have occasional bleeding. *This* put me back on the hook with a few of my patients.

The continuous regimen maintains a favorable effect on CVD risk factors, prevents osteoporosis, provides continuous relief of menopausal symptoms, protects the endometrium, and does not cause growth of uterine fibroids. Using Provera at only 2.5 mg, the progestin side effects are absent or minimal. It works best if you are two to three years beyond your last menstrual period; earlier use is fraught with more breakthrough bleeding.

The continuous regimen is far and away the most popular because most women prefer not to have the regular monthly bleeding of the cyclic methods. Women who are only recently menopausal are more likely to have breakthrough bleeding in the first six months. To accommodate them, they can be initially started on a month of Provera only. This results in a thinner endometrium, with less likelihood of irregular bleeding when the combined continuous regimen is started. For women who are switching from cyclic to continuous HRT, it is usually better to stop hormones altogether for about three months. This avoids the frustrations of irregular bleeding in the initial months.

An unknown about continuous HRT is whether breasts require *cyclic* progestin or not. No studies exist to point in either direction. One other possible negative is that an increasing number of women who have used continuous HRT successfully for many years are getting breakthrough bleeding again—not many, but it is being investigated.

WHEN YOU CAN'T USE ESTROGEN

When estrogen use is contraindicated because of a health problem such as chronic liver disease, past thromboembolism, or an estrogen dependent tumor, several nonestrogen options are available. Likewise, if you just decide you don't want to use estrogen for whatever reason that is important to you, these alternatives could be considered. Those on the following list have been used for hot flashes. None of them plays a role in prevention of CVD, and with the exception of the progestins, none prevents osteoporosis.

+ *Progestin alone* can be used. Provera tablets are taken daily in a dose range of 2.5 mg up to 10–20 mg. It is effective in relieving hot flashes for about 80%–90% of women. In addition, there is a beneficial influence on calcium utilization to help prevent bone loss. In the absence of estrogen, about 1,500 mg of calcium is needed on a daily basis. Assuming your diet provides 500 mg, add a 1,000 mg supplement. Vaginal atrophy is not prevented by progestin, so dryness and painful sex can still occur. Small doses of estrogen cream or the estrogen ring used vaginally can be quite helpful. Estrogen *is* absorbed into your bloodstream through your vagina, so whether or not this could harm your underlying health condition should be thoroughly discussed with your doctor. Provera at the higher dose levels will decrease your good guy HDL cholesterol, therefore lipid profile monitoring is advised. Provera at higher dose levels may also produce some of the disagreeable side effects mentioned above.

+ *Depo-Provera* (depo-medroxyprogesterone acetate, or DMPA) is a long acting form of Provera that also works to control hot flashes in doses of 150 mg injected every three months.

+ *Megace* (megestrol acetate) is another progestin that can control hot flashes. In 10–20 mg doses twice daily, Megace reduces the frequency of hot flashes by about 85%, according to a Mayo Clinic study. It is the only type of progestin approved by the FDA for use in women who have had breast cancer.

+ *Catapres* (clonidine) is a drug used primarily for high blood pressure. It sometimes is effective in relieving hot flashes. It is available in tablets and a transdermal skin patch. The downside to using this drug is that it can lower normal blood pressure and produce dizziness.

+ *Parlodel* (bromocriptine) is a drug that has been used to suppress lactation. It is partially effective in controlling hot flashes. To be effective, Parlodel must be used in high doses and is fraught with side effects such as low blood pressure and dizziness and occasionally with intensely high blood pressure.

+ *Veralipride* is a dopamine antagonist that can inhibit hot flashes in doses of 100 mg daily. Side effects include sore breasts and milk production.

+ *Aldomet* (methyldopa) is a blood pressure medication that will inhibit hot flashes in daily doses of 500–1,000 mg. It may initially cause sedation and drowsiness. Less common side effects can include low blood pressure, slow heart rate, nausea, diarrhea, and gassiness.

- *Bellergal* is an antispasmodic drug used for gastrointestinal problems. It can help some women with their hot flashes, but it can also slow the digestive process and cause blurred vision.
- *Vitamin E* has been reported to be helpful for hot flashes by many users in doses of 400 units per day. It has not been well studied, so good information is not available as to the mechanism of its effect.
- *Sedatives* and *tranquilizers*, if used briefly, can be helpful for hot flashes. Sedatives reduce irritability in the autonomic nervous system, which is the part of your nervous system that controls blood vessel dilation. Tranquilizers exert their influence by suppressing the hypothalamus, which is your body's thermostat. The well-known drawback of both these types of drugs is that they are very habit forming, so long-term use is not wise.
- *Additional alternative therapies* are covered in Chapter 12. Of those listed, *black cohosh* is probably the most effective in controlling hot flashes. It is a vasoconstrictor, meaning it prevents your skin capillaries from dilating and hence, inhibits hot flashes.

The Androgen Story in HRT

The term *androgen* refers to all the male hormones. There are five of them, which you will find listed in Table 11-4. Both sexes make female and male hormones. The essential difference between men and women is that one of these hormones is far and away the dominant hormone. You already know which is dominant in whom, but I'll bet you didn't know that your female hormones are made from male hormones. Yes, it's true. The actual starting point for hormone production is with a cholesterol molecule. It is reconfigured chemically in the *stroma* (core tissue) of your ovaries to testosterone and then converted chemically to an estrogen molecule by the cells of the egg follicles on the surface of your ovaries. After all this, your estrogen goes out to your cellular receptor sites and does all those marvelous female things to which you have become accustomed.

Your ovaries make the first two androgens listed in Table 11-4. Most, but not all, of the testosterone (T) and androstenedione (ASD) is used to make estrogen. Tiny amounts of T and ASD are left over for other uses in your body. Testosterone, the strongest androgen, has important functions in maintaining your sexual desire, keeping your energy level adequate, building bone, maintaining muscles, and promoting a sense of wellness. ASD, a weak androgen, is the source of estrone that is made from your fat cells.

Table 11-4
ANDROGENS
Testosterone (T)
Androstenedione (ASD)
Dehydroepiandrosterone (DHEA)
Dehydroepiandrosterone sulfate (DHEAS)
Dihydrotestosterone (DHT)

ASD, together with another weak androgen, DHEA, is also made in your adrenal glands. When these two reach your ovaries via your bloodstream, they too can be converted to estrogen by the follicle cells.

That's the background information. Now the plot thickens. From puberty to menopause, your body maintains a constant ratio of huge amounts of estrogen to minuscule amounts of testosterone. The ratio begins to change in perimenopause through to menopause as your follicles diminish in number. By the time you have reached menopause, 80%–90% of your ovarian estrogen production is lost because of the reduction in the number of remaining follicles. However, only about 50% of your testosterone production is lost because T is produced in those interior stromal cells, not in your follicles. Both hormones are reduced in amount, but the ratio is now changed.

With less overall testosterone available, you may start experiencing loss of muscle mass, less energy to get through your average frantic day, you are less of a sex bomb than before, and you know that you just don't feel completely well but can't put a finger on why. With your remaining testosterone less overpowered by estrogen, T may start doing malelike things to you: more facial hair, slightly deeper voice, change in body fat distribution from the female pear-shaped concentration about the hips to the male apple-shaped ditribution around the waist. The new estrogen-testosterone balance puts you at higher risk for other unfavorable male problems such as a rising blood pressure, higher cholesterol, and an unfavorable lipid ratio of HDL to LDL.

THAT'S AWFUL. WHAT SHOULD I DO?

If you are noticing both estrogen and testosterone deficiency symptoms, replacement with both hormones has been found to be quite beneficial. Halotestin (*fluoxymesterone*) is the only synthetic androgen tablet available in tablet doses small enough for women. *Methyltestosterone*, formerly the most commonly used synthetic, has fallen into disuse in favor of the better tolerated fluoxymesterone. Methyltestosterone is still available in a tablet combined with estrogen called Estratest. Halotestin and Estratest are in increasingly common use for women on HRT. For the most part, they produce significant improvement in your sense of wellness. One of the most welcome benefits is improved sexual desire and sexual fantasies. Table 11-5 illustrates what dosage effects to expect from androgen use.

For the most part, dosage standards have been based on the needs known for men, and that is far too high for women. For example, a male dose may be 10–50 mg to start and higher after that. For you, 1–2 mg per day or every other day may be all that is needed. It would be rare for you to need more than 5 mg per day. If you should get to that dose level without improvement in symptoms, your total testosterone blood level should be checked before going any higher. If it is in the desirable range, other causes should be

Table 11-5

TESTOSTERONE DOSAGE EFFECTS

Insufficient	Ideal	Excessive
Decreased sexual desire	Normal desire	Above normal sexual desire
Low body energy	Normal energy	Overactiveness
Slowed thinking	Alert	Short attention span
Mild depression	Positive mood	Anxiety, irritability
Fewer dreams	Normal dreams	Aggressive, violent dreams
Thin, dry skin	Normal skin	Acne
Thin, fine hair	Normal hair	Facial hair

investigated as the source of your symptoms. Hypothyroidism, overproduction of prolactin by your pituitary, and depression may all be candidates.

The normal testosterone (T) level for you is 60–90 nannograms per milliliter. It needs to be between 30 and 60 ng/ml to maintain optimal sexual desire. Levels below 20 will put sex very low on your agenda of important things to do. By comparison, the normal T level in men is 300–1,200 ng/ml. His sex drive diminishes when it gets below 500, but this doesn't usually happen in men until their 60s or later. In you, however, a 10–15 ng/ml drop can make an enormous difference because you are sensitive to very small amounts of testosterone.

BUT I DON'T WANT TO LOOK LIKE A PROFESSIONAL WRESTLER

Androgen excess effects are not usually encountered if the total monthly dose is kept in the 50–75 mg range. If higher doses are used, your lipid profile should be monitored because long-term use may lower your good guy HDL. Androgen use must start in low doses, with only gradual increases until the desired effect is achieved. Each of you is different, so a one-dose-for-everyone approach doesn't work.

The myths about male hormone use in women are mostly all negative: more facial hair, acne, bulging muscles, deep voice, and a sex drive that you can't satisfy with a platoon of partners. These things have happened in some degree to women taking androgens, but the adverse effects have always been related to the *dose* and *type* of male hormone used.

HOW DO I TAKE IT?

There are various routes of administration.

♦ The oral tablet is the preferable method for taking testosterone. Natural micronized testosterone from soy beans and Mexican yams is available. It is not made commercially, but it can be obtained from specialty pharmacies listed in Appendix B. Natural testosterone tablets can be dissolved under your tongue; this is an efficient way to get it into your system. Your uterine endometrium is not protected by testosterone so you still need progesterone. Table 11-6 lists the commercially available types of testosterone.

♦ Injections of T have the disadvantage of wide fluctuation in blood levels, from too high after the shot to too low before the next one. This subjects you to many of the unwanted side effects listed in Table 11-5. An advantage of injections is that they bypass your intestinal tract and your liver, thereby sidestepping their inactivation effects. This route avoids any negative effect on HDL.

♦ Pellets placed under your skin are being used by some physicians. They contain 75 mg of T and last for three months. They also bypass the liver and have no effect on HDL. Pellets should only be used after your individual dose requirements have been established by the oral method, because once pellets are placed, you can't take them out.

♦ A skin patch may be a future possibility, but now it is only available for men and is therefore too large a dose.

Table 11-6

COMMERCIAL TETOSTERONE PREPARATIONS

Brand name	Type of hormone	Doses available
(Testosterone only)		
Android-10	Methyltestosterone	10 mg capsules
Halotestin	Fluoxymesterone	2, 5, 10 mg tablets
Depo-Testadiol, Testone LA, Delatest	Testosterone enthanate	100 mg/ml injectable
Depo-Test	Testosterone cypionate	50 mg/ml injectable
(Testosterone-estrogen combinations)		
Estratest	Methyltestosterone Esterified estrogens	2.5 mg 1.25 mg } tablet
Estratest HS (half strength)	Methyltestosterone Esterified estrogens	1.25 mg 0.625 mg } tablet
Depo-Testadiol	Testosterone cypionate Estradiol cypionate	50 mg 2 mg } injectable

Androgen use is a special situation that you may or may not need. If you are experiencing typical testosterone deficiency symptoms, especially a diminished sexual desire, a trial is worthwhile. If androgens fail to improve your symptoms with doses appropriate for women, a higher dose level should not be attempted without a blood level check. If your blood level is normal and your symptoms persist, other causes must be investigated.

DHEA (DEHYDROEPIANDROSTERONE) — THE "FOUNTAIN OF YOUTH"?

This is one of the weak androgens listed in Table 11-4. It is derived from a plant source and is therefore available without prescription. There is a lot of commercial hype about combining DHEA with vitamins and reversing or stopping the aging process. In your body, DHEA is made in your adrenal glands. Some of it circulates in your bloodstream as free DHEA, but most is bonded to a sulfate to become DHEAS. If needed, it can be converted to testosterone.

It has been demonstrated that DHEA reaches its peak level in your body in your late 20s, just like estrogen. Then, it begins a long slow decline for the rest of your life. The steady decline is not affected by menopause as is estrogen, and by your 70s you will have lost about 80% of your DHEA.

Research with laboratory mice and rats produced some surprising results with DHEAS use. It stopped or slowed many age-related events such as diabetes, breast cancer, immune system decline, genetic mutations from carcinogen exposure, and weight gain; the life span of the rats and mice was increased (Schwartz 1995).

In humans, it was observed that the natural decline in DHEA and DHEAS corresponded to the rising risk of CVD in men; in women however the CVD risk was highest in those with the *highest* levels of these androgens. When men and women were given high doses of DHEA and DHEAS, the results differed. On 1,600 mg, men improved their lipoprotein profiles, but it worsened in women, who developed the malelike apple-shaped fat distribution. On smaller 50 mg doses, however, women were noted to have many positive benefits:

✦ improved immune system competence with more protective activity from natural killer cells. This can translate to cancer protection (Araneo 1995)
✦ no decrease in insulin sensitivity which occurs with aging and can result in diabetes (Bates 1995)
✦ better sleep, memory, and mood (Baulieu 1995)

- ✦ beneficial effect in major depression (Wolkowitz 1995)
- ✦ increased energy
- ✦ improved ability to handle stress
- ✦ no weight gain

These are exciting results, especially the prospect of reducing the age-related cancer risks. The studies to date have been small, and a great deal more work is yet to be done before these androgens can be regarded as the elusive fountain of youth. The current FDA stance is that in the absence of large, long-term studies to support the above claims, it will not approve DHEA for any indication. Meanwhile the DHEA craze is on, led by whoever can hawk their DHEA-laced vitamins and food supplements the loudest.

Melatonin and Menopause

The hormone melatonin is produced in tiny amounts by the *pineal* gland in the center of your brain. Melatonin burst onto the health scene in 1995 with all the enthusiasm of a stampede. Available over the counter, it has been promoted as an inexpensive, nontoxic, and nonhabituating sleep medication. In the near future, it has the potential to play an alleviatory role in menopausal sleep disruption and the resulting irritability, short-term memory loss, and fatigue. We know that as FSH rises with menopause, melatonin falls. This has led to speculation that melatonin supplements may be helpful.

This hormone is thought to be an integral part of our biological clock that controls aging. Research has shown that decreasing melatonin production contributes to the aging process at the cellular level. Melatonin decreases heart rate, lowers blood pressure, diminishes digestion, relaxes muscles, and lulls you to sleep. It has the opposite effect of adrenaline, which prepares us for "fight or flight." More of it is produced at night, which accounts for why it is a sleep-inducing drug. Laboratory animals treated with melatonin lived significantly longer lives, with fewer of the diseases associated with aging (heart disease, cancer, diabetes, high blood pressure, cataracts, high cholesterol). It is fun to think that there could be a method for the prevention of age-related diseases, rather than just trying to treat them. So, we need for those melatonin-crazed researchers to keep at it and produce some hard data. Thus far they have not, and for that reason it seems prudent to use this hormone with caution. Britain and France have banned over-the-counter sales of melatonin, while Italy and Denmark have forbidden many promotional advertising claims touting its medical benefits. In our country, it is a nonprescription drug, and the sky's the limit for promoters.

No HRT

A frequently asked and commonly debated question is "Do I really need hormones?" There is little disagreement that HRT will control the symptoms of hormone withdrawal and will improve the odds against developing heart disease, osteoporosis, and endometrial cancer. This leads to the obvious conclusion, for some, that every woman should be on HRT.

On the other hand, other measures can be protective as well. If you have been following a healthy lifestyle since your youth incorporating good nutrition, regular exercise, no smoking, and minimal alcohol consumption, you are likely to arrive at menopause with cardiovascular fitness and a sturdy skeleton. Your personal risk factors for CVD and osteoporosis are low, aside from any family-related risks. Assuming you continue this lifestyle after menopause, plus some additions such as extra calcium and more attention to low fat intake, then hormone replacement may not be necessary for you. HRT for you would be an adjunct rather than a preventive treatment—an option as opposed to a necessity. Adjunctive use of HRT is still an advantage, since the data show that a healthy lifestyle plus hormone use is more protective than either of them alone.

If your decision is not to use hormone replacement in any fashion, consider having an annual checkup of your uterine lining and a periodic DEXA scan for evidence of osteoporosis. Your chances of getting an endometrial cancer are increased if you are not using a progestin, but there are steps you can take to monitor that possibility. Have an annual vaginal ultrasound scan. If your endometrium is less than 5 mm in depth, nothing further need be done for a year. Ultrasound is harmless, but at $150 to $200 a pop, it's rather expensive. If your endometrium measures over 5 mm, a biopsy will tell you what is going on. Benign thickening, called hyperplasia, can be reverted to normal with a course of progestin.

Summing Up

Aging is an immutable fact of life; hormones will not prevent it. That's just the way it is. Some of the disagreeable symptoms that result from menopause can be controlled or muted, and several disabling or life threatening problems can be avoided. There is little question that women who suffer the symptoms of hormone depletion should be relieved of them if possible. Estrogen is a slam-dunk to do it, for most. In addition, there is no longer any scientific dispute that estrogen will substantially prevent the long-term disabilities associated with osteoporosis and dramatically reduce the risk of cardiovascular disease. Progestins protect the endometrium. Androgens improve your sense of well-being and sexual desire.

The bottom line regarding HRT is that virtually every recent and respected scientific study has shown it to be remarkably safe and effective. In view of this, I feel strongly that all women in midlife should be told of these potential benefits, as well as the drawbacks, and be offered hormone replacement therapy. The U.S. Food and Drug Administration Advisory Committee agrees; it unanimously recommended that all women who *can* take estrogen should consider it at menopause.

As far as how long you should take HRT, the answer is, as long as you desire the benefits. The decision to use HRT or decline it belongs to each woman. It should be based on your having adequate information, on your trust in your health adviser, and on your own intellectual perceptions and intuitive feelings.

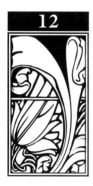

12

ALTERNATIVE THERAPIES

The symptoms generated by hormone depletion can be improved for some by using a variety of treatments that steer clear of Western medicine's hormone therapy course. Candidates for these alternatives tend to be women who must not take estrogen for health reasons, women who decline HRT for philosophical reasons, and women who have responded poorly to HRT (sore breasts, irregular bleeding, depression, etc.). At this point in time, many of these alternatives are not mainstream therapies because of the lack of good scientific evidence confirming their safety and effectiveness. The U.S. Food & Drug Administration (FDA) has been essentially silent on this subject, but that is not necessarily a damning stance. The FDA has not approved Provera for use in menopause either, but the evidence for its efficacy is overwhelming, so we in the medical community prescribe it. With increasing interest in alternative medicine, and growing use by the public, appropriate studies are being done. Many HMOs are now beginning to recognize and cover these therapies.

The following pages will cover homeopathy, Chinese herbal medicine, acupuncture, holistic medicine, and a brief reference to mind/body medicine. As is true with all medical practices, these therapies are not the answer for everyone. The substances used are mostly naturally occurring plant and animal derivatives, which are available without a prescription. The scientific warning when using these remedies is that the exact dose (in milligrams) of their active ingredients is not always known; sometimes the active ingredient itself is not known, or the physiological effect of the active ingredient is not clear. Nevertheless, many people are helped by them, and there is no denying it. A discussion of these various techniques and treatments is appropriate and necessary to a fair presentation of the subject of menopausal management.

Homeopathy

This medical discipline was founded in the late 1700s by Samuel Hahnemann, a German physician and chemist (Ullman 1991). It is accepted by 40%–50% of English, Dutch, and French physicians as useful and effective care (Bouchayer 1990). The majority of European physicians do not regard homeopathy as primary care. Its premise is similar to that of mind/body medicine, in which the mind and body are inseparable and mutually dependent. Homeopathy presupposes that if symptoms are displayed by the body, they are a signal that the mind/body is trying to heal itself or to adapt to an altered milieu. For example, fever is a symptom of infection, a mood change is a response to a stressor, hot flashes are a symptom of hormone depletion. In this respect, homeopathy shares these views with traditional, Western medical beliefs.

The difference between homeopathic care and allopathic (traditional) care is in the approach to treatment. The allopathic model for treatment of disease involves producing a condition incompatible with the sources of the disease. An example would be use of an antibiotic to combat infection. In contrast, homeopathic remedies involve the prescribing of very tiny amounts of substances which, if given in large amounts, would produce the very symptom of which you are complaining. The prescribed substance is diluted to hundredths or thousandths of the original strength and then taken a few drops at a time. The theory is that these minuscule doses will stimulate your body's defenses to mount an attack against whatever is producing the offensive symptoms, by first exaggerating those very symptoms. Allergists use this same principle in desensitizing people. They give tiny but increasing doses of whatever you are allergic to, until you have built up sufficient antibodies to be protected. A homeopathic remedy is not considered to be working if you do not feel an initial increase in your complaint. Two or three remedies may be tried before finding the correct one. Experienced homeopaths do not generally use more than one remedy at a time. A successful remedy for one person may be utterly useless for another with exactly the same problem. The substance prescribed is not regarded as having cured you, because of the extremely small amounts you received. Your improvement is regarded to have come from your body's natural defenses having been nudged by the homeopathic remedy to cause healing.

Two types of remedies exist:

1. Constitutional. This type is used to treat the entire person, meaning physical and psychological symptoms, as well as abnormal personality variants.
2. Nonconstitutional. These remedies are oriented toward specific symptoms.

Initial interviews with a homeopathic practitioner are characteristically quite extensive. The practitioner is interested in all aspects of your life: age, general health, symptoms, relationships with spouse, family, and others, occupation, education, diet, moods, and many other external and internal factors affecting your life. By combining knowledge of your complaint with lifestyle factors that may be playing a role, a remedy is selected. All of the remedy substances are naturally occurring in plant or animal life. Improvement is rarely immediate and, indeed, may require several weeks or months. Practitioners emphasize that a patient must be committed to this mode of treatment to improve chances of success, because homeopathic healing is a process, as opposed to a single visit and a cure. It may take six months to two years to achieve the stated goal of healing you on the mental, physical, and emotional levels. Relief of your menopausal symptoms may be achieved, but there is no hard scientific proof that homeopathic remedies will protect you against the two major post-menopausal threats: osteoporosis and cardiovascular disease.

Homeopathists urge that self-treatment not be undertaken, since a broad understanding of the substances used is necessary for success. A significant number of homeopathists are medical doctors, while some are nurses and acupuncturists. All are licensed health practitioners. No specific training is required to prescribe homeopathic remedies. The level of expertise varies widely. This may cause disappointing results for you, so question the practitioner you consult closely regarding their experience with menopausal symptoms and effectiveness of treatment.

To locate a homeopathic practitioner, contact the

National Center for Homeopathy
810 North Fairfax, #306
Alexandria, VA 22314
(703) 548-7790

Chinese Herbal Medicine and Acupuncture

When Western medicine was having its beginnings, Chinese herbal medicine had already been in existence over 3,000 years. Its premise is that the body must be in harmony with the world around it at all stages of life, if good health is to be enjoyed (Bienfield 1991). Chinese herbal practitioners have identified in the human body 12 channels of energy flow between five energy centers located in your kidneys, liver, lungs, heart, and spleen. Each channel of energy flow has its own distinctive pulse. By monitoring these pulses, health status is assessed.

The Chinese term for this energy is *Qi* (pronounced chee). Chinese medicine incorporates the belief that each of us is born with a finite amount of Qi, which can be depleted by various events and problems in life. This exposes us to greater risk of disease. Our obligation in maintaining good health is to protect our Qi stores and replenish them when necessary. If the flow of Qi is blocked or restricted, or if you have too much Qi or too little, then the flow through these 12 channels is out of balance, and your exposure to disease is increased.

Qi must be replenished when you are in times of stress, or diseased, or in a transition. This is accomplished by the use of herbs, by acupuncture, by relaxation techniques, and by diet. The herbs prescribed are those that target the particular organ system perceived to be out of balance and thus the source of your symptoms. Often a mixture of herbs is brewed into a tea, or a liquid extract may be prepared for direct ingestion. The herbs can be quite potent in many instances. Though self-treatment is widely available through health food stores, it is urged that you use Chinese herbs only under the direction of an experienced practitioner.

The 12 energy channels are like a grid; they intersect at various points in your body. It is believed that these intersections are the sites where energy flow alterations occur. This forms the basis for acupuncture treatment. By inserting tiny needles at known locations, neurotransmitters are released, causing energy flow to be slowed or enhanced, or even transferred from one channel to another, to aid a faltering organ system. Electrical stimulation and massage of the appropriate points are also used.

One of the 12 channels is called *the three healers*. This channel is said to harmonize and integrate the three metabolic systems of respiration, digestion, and elimination. Chinese herbal practitioners often focus on the three healers to control menstrual irregularity and other menopausal symptoms through the use of herbal mixtures and acupuncture.

An organization in North Carolina can be contacted for more information and referral to a Chinese medical practitioner in your area:

AAAOM Referrals
4101 Lake Boone Trail #201
Raleigh, NC 27607-6518
(919) 787-5181

Holistic Medicine

Holistic medicine is also referred to as *alternative* or *complimentary medicine*. It is another variation of the healing arts, practiced by licensed physicians. It is patient-centered, as opposed to disease-centered, its basic premise being that all medical disciplines (Western, Eastern; traditional, alternative) can be integrated and used to compliment each other. The holistic approach is to stress nontoxic and noninvasive treatments such as herbal medicine, nutritional therapy, acupuncture, stress management (meditation, yoga, prayer, hypnotism), and homeopathy. When deemed necessary, Western techniques are employed such as X ray, laboratory testing, prescription medicines, and surgery. Some of the nonconventional therapies of holistic medicine such as vitamin megadoses and nutritional management of disease are receiving more serious scientific attention, and they are emerging as conventional, mainstream therapy.

Mind/Body Medicine

The thread running through all of the above alternative treatment disciplines is what is being referred to as mind/body medicine. A full explanation of this fascinating concept is beyond the scope of this book. For those of you who are genuinely interested, get a copy of *Quantum Healing* by Deepak Chopra, M.D. In it you will find an extraordinary, new, nonorthodox, and non-Western approach to healing. The essence of mind/body medicine is that each of us is a package of intelligence that happens to be contained in a body. All cells of the body are in constant communication with each other by chemicals called neurotransmitters. Hormones are good examples. Everything is under the command and control of the intelligence pool, the mind. In this sense, *mind* means more than just the brain and the nervous system; mind includes the intelligence that resides in each of the trillions of cells of the entire body. If something goes wrong, such as a certain cell turning into a cancer cell, the intelligence network is immediately aware of it and healing is set in motion. It is possible that we cure ourselves of cancer hundreds of times this way, but these healing commands can get overwhelmed by certain illnesses, such as cancer or infection, and lose the battle. The challenge in mind/body medicine is to tap into this intelligence deliberately and consciously, rather than have it working at the subconscious level, where it normally operates. It follows that this "mind" we all possess would be a *very* efficient healer with its huge database and unlimited capacity to fashion defenses to disease. It could make traditional and alternative medical strategies seem very crude. Fascinating concept.

Substances Utilized

If you opt for nonhormonal treatment, you will no doubt be bumping into a number of unfamiliar names and substances. The following is a listing of a few of the more commonly advocated remedies for menopausal symptoms. Note that while symptomatic relief is widely claimed by prescriber and patient alike, none of these remedies has been shown to prevent postmenopausal cardiovascular disease—the 900-pound gorilla.

+ *Ginseng.* This Chinese herb is commonly used for menopausal complaints. The *panax* variety from China or Korea, as opposed to Siberian or American ginseng, is preferred. It is used to treat temperature imbalance such as hot flashes; however, depression and fatigue may also be helped, since it is basically a stimulant. Ginseng has estrogenic properties that may cause uterine bleeding in postmenopausal women. Unopposed estrogen precautions are advised. It should be avoided, or used with great caution, by women who have had breast cancer or who have risk factors for endometrial cancer. Good ginseng is very expensive.
+ *Dong quai.* This is an herb with strong estrogenic effect because it contains high amounts of *phytosterols.* Phytosterols are not really hormones, but they provide precursor chemicals from which your body can manufacture hormones. Usually, large doses are prescribed if an estrogenic effect is desired. Dong quai is beneficial for hot flashes because it is a vasoconstrictor: It prevents blood vessels from dilating, therefore, large quantities of blood can't be brought to the surface vessels in your skin, and you get fewer hot flashes. If you are not on a progestin but *are* on dong quai, you are essentially using unopposed estrogen. In this situation, you would be well advised to have your endometrium monitored annually with an ultrasound scan, and a biopsy if indicated. Breast cancer patients should avoid dong quai. Phytosterol use is quite controversial, as you might expect.
+ *Black cohosh.* This is an herb used by Native Americans for menstrual cramps. It is thought to have substances that relieve pain and act as sedatives. There is sufficient estrogenic activity to improve hot flashes, diminish vaginal atrophy, and even can lower the FSH produced by your pituitary gland. Black cohosh is also a vasoconstrictor, which accounts in part for improved hot flashes. In a double blind study (aka randomized clinical trial) of hot flash control, black cohosh was compared with 0.625 mg of conjugated estrogen and with a placebo. Black cohosh was found superior to both Premarin and the placebo for control of hot flashes and other estrogen deficiency symptoms.

Because no studies exist on the risk for endometrial cancer with this herb, it is recommended that it be used no longer than three to six months (Tyler 1997). It is now known that as little as six months of unopposed estrogen increases the risk of endometrial cancer fourfold, and the increased risk lingers for several years.

✦ *Evening primrose oil.* This is a fatty acid derived from high-fat fish such as tuna, salmon, mackerel, and rainbow trout. It also comes from the seed oils of sunflower, sesame, corn, wheat germ, and safflower plants. Evening primrose oil is said to improve function of the brain, eyes, adrenal glands, and reproductive organs by developing a more effective cell membrane, where fatty acids are essential. It has been widely used for menstrual cramps, vaginal dryness, and PMS. Several placebo controlled studies have shown it does not benefit PMS more than a placebo. It does not help hot flashes but may delay their onset. Unopposed estrogen precautions are advisable.

✦ *Lachesis.* A homeopathic remedy derived from the venom of the American bushmaster snake, it is used for women who are characterized as overbearing and demanding and have fits of rage or jealousy, migraines, and strong libidos.

✦ *Pulsatilla.* Made from the windflower, this homeopathic remedy is used for women who are shy and nonassertive, weep easily, lack energy, have low libidos, but have an increased need for love and acceptance.

✦ *Sepia.* One of the most commonly used homeopathic remedies for menopause, it is derived from the inky secretions of the cuttlefish. It is said to be helpful for those who feel tired and run down, have low sex drives, are often irritable, and have dryness of the eyes, mouth, and vagina.

✦ *Nux vomica.* This homeopathic remedy made from the poison nut helps relieve backache and nausea and reduce frequent awakening during the night, perfectionistic tendencies, and chronic anger.

✦ *Bioflavinoids.* More than 400 different types exist, all somewhat differing in their effects. They are derived from soy beans, oriental spices, green tea, citrus fruits, and citrus rinds. Japanese women, who have very few menopausal symptoms, consume about 5,000 mg of bioflavinoids daily. The average American diet contains 800–1,000 mg (Aldercreutz 1992). They are mildly estrogenic and help somewhat with hot flashes.

There are many other products available and used to treat menopausal symptoms including agnus castus, red sage, beth root, damiana, sarsaparilla, cramp bark, red raspberry leaves, golden seal, licorice root, and spearmint. For those that are estrogenic, it is important to keep in mind that they carry the same potential for complication as unopposed estrogen replacement therapy. The prescribing practitioner, as well as the woman who uses these therapies, must have a clear understanding of the active ingredient and what to look for, if unintended results are to be avoided. A good example of a major unanswered question is, Does long-term use result in more endometrial cancer? The paucity of research to evaluate the true safety, effectiveness, and purity of these substances justifies caution in their use. It is encouraging that the National Institutes of Health have recently opened the Office for Alternative Medicine. Hopefully, this will result in broader understanding and acceptance when adequate studies are completed.

Summing Up

About 70%–80% of menopausal American women do not use hormone replacement. With the current public perception that hormone replacement is somehow bad for you, it is not surprising that other options are sought by the large majority of hormone nonusers. This has been enhanced in recent years by an emerging antagonism toward practitioners of Western medicine and a distrust for Western medicines. The women who are turning away from Western science have been wholeheartedly accepted by alternative medical practitioners. As a result, egregious turf battles have been waged by practitioners from both sides with mutual condemnation of the opposing discipline. The unfortunate consequence has been an either-or mind-set by health providers and health care recipients alike. The loser in this polarization is you. Both traditional and alternative medical practices can benefit you. If you decide to embrace one and exclude the other, you may be denying yourself an important and necessary service. Fortunately, evidence is beginning to emerge that the middle ground is being sought. Each of these disciplines has much to offer toward the goal of wellness, as well as to each other.

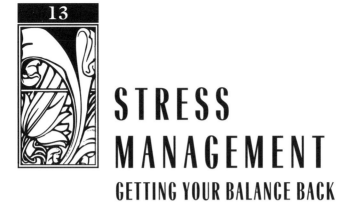

STRESS MANAGEMENT
GETTING YOUR BALANCE BACK

Stress is not age related. All of us experience stress from a huge variety of sources throughout life. It is just part of living. Stress is a common accompaniment of the climacteric years. It derives not only from the daunting symptoms and threatening health problems of perimenopause and menopause, but also from the negative cultural perception that menopausal women should relegate themselves to the back of life's bus. Stress control is therefore an important aspect of menopausal management. It is known that chronic stress can have an adverse impact on many aspects of your health and result in common disorders of the cardiovascular and respiratory systems, as well as insomnia, arthritis, chronic pain, depression, and even cancer. Stress suppresses your immune system, decreasing its ability to ward off a variety of infections. In this chapter you will learn about how stress unbalances your body both physiologically and psychologically and which mechanisms your body employs to restore the balance. A variety of stress management techniques of proven effectiveness are outlined.

Stress Defined

Stress is a very commonly employed word in our culture. It is used to describe everything from emotional disturbance to concrete construction techniques. Stress results from change in the biological, psychological, environmental, or social spheres of our lives. It can arise either internally or externally. The change can be physical or emotional, real or imagined. Change becomes stressful if we perceive it as a threat and if we perceive that we may not be able to cope with it. At that point, the situation has exceeded our comfort level and generated unpleasant emotions such as anger, fear, and anxiety (ACOG 1990).

Stress demands of us that we make some accommodation to it. Should our compensating reaction to a stressor be inadequate or inappropriate, it can give rise to a variety of physical and emotional disorders. In the past, the demanded change tended to be regarded positively as an opportunity or a stimulus to emotional and intellectual growth: "My boss is really piling the work onto me, but I'm going to be much more skillful after I have mastered it." A real Pollyanna, right? A typical response of today would be: "What a slave driver. I can't take it anymore. Does he think I am some kind of robot?" The latter type of response represents the more recent change in our culture that has come to regard stress in largely negative terms.

STRESS IS GOOD FOR YOU

There are some positive aspects of stress. While it is true that heavy stress can overwhelm your coping abilities and adversely affect you, some stress is necessary for a fulfilling life. Stress fertilizes your creativity. Successfully coping with a stressful situation challenges your intellect and emotions. You benefit mentally and physically by positively adapting to a challenge, not by avoiding it or crumbling when faced by it. A life without stress would be boring indeed.

Molecular biologist Stuart Kauffman is an expert in the science of *complex adaptive systems*. This term describes any system that interacts with, adapts to, and evolves with its surroundings. A living cell is a complex adaptive system; so is a rainforest, a business, or a national economy. *You* are a complex adaptive system. Studies have shown living systems function at their most robust and efficient level when they are positioned at the edge of disarray in the narrow space between stability and chaos. Indeed, our highest level of functioning is achieved in such an atmosphere (Yerkes & Dodson 1989). This sounds like a pressure cooker, but it has been observed that humans have the fullest exchange of useful information and the most productive interactions when poised on the precipice of disorder. For example, have you ever noticed how a somewhat untidy office is the most productive one? Have you observed that seemingly disorganized and rollicking families are often the happiest? The point of this is that we need variation and change to reach our fullest potential. They are stressful, but adapting to variation and change is our means to a fulfilling and satisfying life. So, complete avoidance of stress is not healthy for any of us.

STRESS-HARDINESS

Psychologist Suzanne Kobasa has observed that some people adapt to stress better and more naturally than others. They have "stress-hardy" personalities. With positive stress-coping abilities they are capable of experiencing stress without sustaining the typical negative mental and physical effects. Such people are characterized by three important attitudes toward life's vagaries: a sense of control of their life, an acceptance of change as a challenge rather than a threat, and a sense of commitment to be involved in their family, their work, and life generally. Stress-hardy people tend to take control of their lives as opposed to passively accepting whatever fate brings them. They regard challenges as opportunities for growth and learning rather than threats to be avoided or escaped. When confronted by a stressful situation, they embrace it, explore the possibilities of resolving the conflict and then become involved in problem solving. Stress-hardy people are Olympic-class copers. The other end of the spectrum is represented by people who respond to stress passively with an attitude of helplessness; this is known as regressive coping. Most of us are somewhere in between.

Kobasa refers to the personal characteristics of control, challenge, and commitment as the "three Cs." Dr. Herbert Benson believes there is a fourth C—closeness. It is based on the observation that people who have good relationships and social support are more stress-hardy than those who feel isolated from personal contact. If "four C" people also incorporate regular exercise and a healthy diet into their lives, their zest for living is improved and their incidence of illness is markedly reduced (Benson 1992).

STRESS IN ACTION IN YOUR BODY

Stress upsets your homeostasis, meaning your steady state. Homeostasis is a constantly changing balance in the physiological, psychological, and social spheres of our lives. The balance is maintained in a relatively steady state by ongoing minor adjustments at the biochemical, cellular, organ-system, psychological, interpersonal, and social levels of our functioning (Chrouso & Gold 1992). Stressors, both external and internal, are always confronting us and threatening to put our homeostasis out of balance. If the stressor does upset the balance, the resulting disharmony is, you guessed it, stress. It can manifest itself in all of the aforementioned function levels.

PHYSIOLOGICAL RESPONSE TO STRESS

Physiological responses to stress involve automatic chemical changes such as an adrenaline surge, which increases arousal, vigilance, and attention. This prepares us to meet a perceived aggressive challenge, whether it be even more demands by the boss, a crisis with a family member, or a charge by an enraged rhinoceros. Don't you just hate it when you're being charged by a rhinoceros? This physiological response to stress is called the *fight or flight response*. It is a profound, innate, and involuntary reaction that occurs whenever we are threatened, whether the threat is real or imagined. It is mediated by the hypothalamus gland in the brain, which signals the sympathetic nervous system to release stress hormones. This served our ancient ancestors well when they were confronted by a snarling saber-toothed tiger. It still works for us in modern society, as when we are faced with emergencies like an aggressive taxi driver who objects to our being in a crosswalk. Today, however, we do not often face life-threatening emergencies like primitive humankind did. Really now, how long has it been since you were charged by an enraged rhinoceros? Our problem is that the fight or flight response cannot distinguish between a serious threat and the everyday stresses of contemporary life. We respond the same to being late for an appointment as to a taxi driver bearing down on us with a blaring horn.

On our honeymoon, Toria and I went to Bora Bora. After dinner one night we watched with morbid fascination the fearsome moray eels they had penned up at the restaurant. Later, while we sat in the darkness on a bench at the end of a long dock and listened to local native villagers singing, a cat unexpectedly jumped up on Toria's lap. Her first illogical thought was that she was being attacked by one of those ugly eels, and she jumped about two feet straight up. She wasn't ready for fight, but she sure was prepared for flight. Her stress was to an imagined threat, but her body's primal response was just as genuine as if that furry creature in her lap were the eel.

The point I am coming to is that we are all confronted by stressors of modern living. Most of the time it is inappropriate for us to either fight or flee. The long-term effect of these repeated fight or flight responses may lead to permanent and harmful physiological effects on our bodies. Stress hormones accelerate the pulse rate, raise blood pressure, speed up breathing, tense muscles, and increase metabolism. In addition, cortisol release by the adrenal glands raises cholesterol and triglyceride blood levels as an energy source, keeps blood sugar levels high, which risks diabetes from insulin exhaustion, retains sodium to keep blood pressure elevated for a perceived emergency, and suppresses the immune system. It is easy to see that if this situation is revisited too frequently, there can be permanent damage. Therefore it is important to find ways to control the harmful effects of this primitive physiological response in order to neutralize the negative effects of stress on our health and well-being.

PSYCHOLOGICAL RESPONSE

Restoring homeostasis by psychological means involves what psychologists and psychiatrists call *defense mechanisms*. These are relatively automatic mental maneuvers that modulate and control the intensity of our emotional response to the stressor, so that behavior in dealing with it is appropriate. This is called coping. It may be judged by you and others as good coping or poor coping. The magnitude of the stressor's threat varies widely from one person to the next, depending on what the stressor means to an individual. Poor coping is a tag that is frequently hung on a person who uses immature defenses such as

Denial: "I can't understand why I'm a size 18. I eat like a bird."

or

Projection: "If the boss hadn't piled all that extra work on me,

I wouldn't have driven this ax through the computer."

Poor coping often leads to social changes, called maladjustment, as well as to true psychological illness such as depression. So, what to do? First, learn how to recognize stress.

Recognizing Stress

It is often easier to recognize the symptoms of stress than the source of it. The symptoms may be emotional, physical, behavioral, or cognitive—or all of the above. Table 13-1 lists some of the most typical symptoms.

These are readily identifiable changes, and it should be easy to recognize those that are typical of your stress responses. When it comes to naming the source of stress, some of them are obvious such as a relationship crisis, loss of a family member, divorce, unemployment, or a new job. Some aren't so obvious. For example, there are numerous biological changes that may occur

Table 13-1
SYMPTOMS OF STRESS

Emotional	Physical	Behavioral	Cognitive
Anxiety	Rapid heart rate	Critical of others	Forgetful
Nervousness	Restless	Can't get things done	Can't make decisions
Anger, acute or chronic	Headaches	Bossy with others	Fuzzy thinking
Irritable, on edge	Stomachaches	Overeating	Creativity diminished
Loneliness	Insomnia	Excess smoking	Sense of humor lost
Boredom with life	Sweaty palms	Overuse of alcohol	Constant worry
Feel pressured	Fatigue	Neglect of personal habits	Trouble concentrating
Fearfulness	Breathlessness	Decreased sexual desire	
Crying	Tension in neck and shoulders		
Unexplained sadness			

during your transitional years which may be sources of stress. Symptoms of estrogen decline may represent a few of them. Other biological changes unrelated to hormones are graying of your hair, the appearance of wrinkles, or declining energy. It may be that you do not deem any one of these biological changes as a stressor, but you nevertheless feel stressed. So, what could it be? If it turns out that the aging process itself is threatening to you, they may collectively be the source of your stress. So, finding the source can sometimes require some expert help. Once recognized, you are in a much better position to deal effectively with them and learn coping skills.

Stress Management Techniques

Menopausal changes, as well as even the threat of them, are definite stressors for many women. A variety of stress management techniques using behavioral modification methods are now in widespread use. In *The Wellness Book*, Benson and Stuart have advocated a *relaxation response*. This is a counterbalancing mechanism to the fight or flight response. Where the primitive fight or flight is an automatic reaction, the relaxation response is an inborn set of physiological changes that can be evoked consciously and voluntarily. It can be learned and practiced effectively.

If practiced regularly, the relaxation response is a state of rest that can have lasting effects. It involves using the image of "letting go." Physically, it means releasing tension from muscles. Emotionally, it means cultivating an attitude of greater equanimity. Mentally, it involves letting go of troubling, worrisome thoughts. To accomplish the relaxation response, two basic components are involved:

1. a mental focusing device, such as monitoring your breathing, repeating a word, phrase, prayer, or sound, or use of a repetitive muscular activity to help shift your mind away from everyday thoughts or concerns
2. a passive attitude toward distracting thoughts. This means gently directing you mind back to the exercise whenever outside or irrelevant thoughts intrude

The steps to accomplish the relaxation response are

+ pick a focus word, phrase, image, or prayer. It can be a neutral word like *peace* or *love* or a number. It can be a phrase from your personal belief system like *The Lord is my shepherd*, or *shalom*, or *Allah*
+ sit in a comfortable position in quiet surroundings
+ close your eyes

+ relax your muscles
+ breathe slowly, and as you do, repeat your focus word or phrase each time you exhale. It is important that you do "diaphragm breathing," which is deeper, rather than "chest breathing," which is more shallow
+ assume a passive attitude. Don't be concerned with how well you are doing. When extraneous thoughts intrude, just say to yourself "Oh well," and resume your focus word or phrase
+ continue the exercise for 10–20 minutes
+ do the exercise one or two times a day

There are a number of behavioral modification techniques involving mental focusing that can be used to elicit the relaxation response. All of them involve the two basic components of repetition of a focus word or phrase and passive disregard of everyday thoughts. The following is a discussion of a few that can prove useful (Girdano 1993).

+ *Deep muscle relaxation* or *progressive muscle relaxation*. This technique has two components. The first is to take slow, deep breaths and control the rhythm of your breathing. This step, in itself, is remarkably relaxing in only a few minutes and is the best in dealing with hot flashes. Secondly, you alternately tense and relax muscle groups throughout your body. This needs to be a systematic progression through your whole body: feet, calves, thighs, buttocks, back, hands, arms, neck, face. It is hard to do this sort of thing at the office, so plan some "alone" time when you can lie down or be comfortably seated and do it. Progression through the entire body takes about 15 minutes.
+ *Visual imagery.* Use deep breathing here, also, but combine it with the memory of some event in your life when you experienced complete relaxation or profound joy. Think about the details of it, the place where it happened, the physical surroundings, how it felt, how it smelled, how you were dressed, what your feelings were. The relaxing effect can be exquisite. For some, it is difficult to do this, so guided imagery can be helpful. Here you are directed to conjure an image by a group leader or by listening to a tape.
+ *Meditation.* This is a method of intense and totally focused concentration. Once again, follow the deep relaxation steps first; then, close your eyes while concentrating on a focus word or phrase, which you repeat over and over again. There is more to it than this, of course, but that is the beginning. Meditation is greatly underestimated in Western cultures, but it produces positive effects for many ailments. Meditation is best learned by direct instruction rather than reading about it in a manual. Many medical centers and HMOs have stress

reduction clinics where this technique can be learned. A good source for audio tapes on meditation is

Jon Kabat-Zinn, Ph.D.
Massachusetts Medical Center
Stress Reduction Clinic
Lexington, MA 02173

✦ *Biofeedback.* In this technique, you are connected to a machine that monitors your heart rate, blood pressure, and skin responses. In this manner, it measures relaxation, or the lack of it. To demonstrate to you what stress looks like on the tracing, you might be asked to do something difficult like reciting the alphabet backward skipping every other letter. That would make me crazy. This produces a stress response that can be readily seen. Then you might be directed to think of something in your past that you regarded as peaceful or serene. The tracing becomes dramatically different from that of the stress response. By building on this newfound method of control, you teach yourself how to relax. Biofeedback is an excellent technique from which anyone can benefit, but it is not as effective in controlling hot flashes as deep breathing.

✦ *Short-term psychotherapy.* This is a less structured and more personalized method for stress management. A major premise of stress management is to first identify the stressor; this is sometimes not as easy as it sounds. Psychotherapy for stress is probably best handled by psychologists whose expertise is in behavioral problems, rather than by psychiatrists whose expertise is mental illness.

Other stress management techniques include massage, acupuncture, yoga, self-hypnosis, stretching, prayer, music, self-help groups, and humor.

Good nutrition and adequate exercise are the topics of the next chapter; each has a role to play in stress management. If you are being stressed by any source, your metabolic rate is increased, and you need more calories—within reason of course. (I am not advocating that you start eating with both hands when you are tense.) Exercise is a very dependable way to diminish stress, especially if it is vigorous. During aerobic exercise beta-endorphins are released; these hormones cause a "high" feeling, followed by an excellent relaxation of your body and your mind.

Don't Get Stressed by Stress Management

All of the above can be beneficial, but it should go without saying that stress management should not itself be stressful. If you get hell-bent on controlling your stress by one means or another, it can turn out to be counterproductive. You become too preoccupied, too rigid, and more stressed. Just the attitude that you are attempting to take control in managing stress is helpful in itself, so making small changes makes more sense than trying to reorganize your entire life in one fell swoop.

Try to be flexible, and avoid the mental trap where you convince yourself that if you are not totally successful in your efforts, then you have totally failed. Superwoman puts herself to this challenge all the time as she copes with raising children, running a household, holding a job, and relating to her spouse, parents, and friends. Keeping all the balls in the air is exhilarating for her, but if one of them drops, she is very self-critical. Better to ask yourself, What is the worst that could happen if I do not accomplish each and every task I have set for myself? The house might still need dusting tomorrow, but it won't be a hog wallow. My family won't starve if they have leftovers tonight. The PTA won't fold if I don't attend tonight's meeting. My job won't implode if I take a three-day weekend. So, what the hell? You will find that very few things are as important as you had originally thought if you ask yourself, What is the worst that could happen? (Landau, 1994).

Two More Stress Managers

What do you suppose laughter and religion have in common? Stress relief. Laughter works both physiologically and psychologically to reduce and relieve stress. It lowers blood pressure, relaxes tense muscles, and puts more oxygen into your system. So tell some jokes, or at least listen to them. When you hear a new joke, try to remember it and tell it to others with your own embellishments. Read humorous books or magazines. See a funny movie. Ever notice how much more you laugh at a funny movie in the theater than if you see it at home on the VCR? Laughter is infectious. Just listening to how others laugh is funny in itself. Laughter has a unique ability to defuse a confrontation. Victor Borge once observed, "Laughter is the shortest distance between two people."

Health humorist Larry Wilde likens a sense of humor to a first-aid kit that you carry with you at all times. It is available at a moment's notice to improve your mood, defuse a confrontation, lower your blood pressure, and relieve your anxiety. He has a five-point plan for improving your health and your life with laughter.

1. Laugh out loud. Physically laughing, as opposed to just grinning or thinking about it, is better for you. It improves your circulation, increases your oxygenation, lowers your blood pressure, and even has a positive influence on your immune system. Maybe laughter and

longevity go hand-in-hand. George Burns made it to 100, and fellow comedians Bob Hope and Milton Berle are well into advanced age.

2. Laugh at yourself. At its roots, laughter is an expression of love and esteem. If you can laugh at your own faults, you basically like yourself and have a healthy self-esteem. Abraham Lincoln, never known as a handsome man, made this comment when he was accused by a detractor of being two-faced: "If I had two faces, would I be showing you this one?" Abe was comfortable with himself.

3. Maintain a lighthearted attitude. Attitude is a choice you make in any situation, so why not choose to be upbeat? A joyful spirit helps control stress, defuses resentment, improves relationships, and makes you a more productive worker. When things are tense, take a 10-minute humor break. Open a joke book or listen to a tape, and then see how smoothly things go afterward. A lighthearted attitude helped an elderly clergyman get through an awkward moment on an elevator when the door opened and a beautiful young woman stepped in totally nude. After an uncomfortable second or two he said, "I like your outfit. My wife has one just like it. Of course, yours fits better."

4. Find something funny every day. Some days it may be a tough search. Life is like that. Maybe it will be only a cartoon in a magazine, but find something. Larry Wilde suggested to an audience of senior citizens, "Maybe you just need to undress and look at yourself in a mirror." That brought the house down with an avalanche of chortles and guffaws.

5. Find the funny side of life, even when you are up to your neck in alligators. It's just as easy to laugh as to cry. When everything has seemingly turned grim, it is not inappropriate to resort to humor. When comedian Jack Benny was on his deathbed, his friends, writers, and family were gathered, and they recalled with mirth their many, many humorous times together. A famous humorist wrote that just as life does not cease to be funny when we die, life does not cease to be serious when we laugh.

A good sense of humor makes coping with stress much more successful. By midlife, your wagon wheel has been through enough ruts that you can look back on them, and on life in general, with a bit of a grin. More of life seems funny by midlife, although I will agree that it isn't *all* just a big hoot. Still, laughter is good for you. It doesn't cost a dime; it's tax-free, cholesterol free, nonfattening, and nontoxic. Humorist Josh Billings said, "There ain't much fun in medicine, but there's a heck of a lot of medicine in fun." So, don't leave home without it.

As for religion, most people by midlife will benefit from a commitment to a formal religion, a deeply felt set of values and beliefs, a sense of spirituality, and a devotion to humanitarianism (Benson 1984). By this time in life, most of us are becoming aware of our own mortality by having experienced personal health problems or by realizing that our parents are near the end of life or already gone. Spirituality helps to confront these realities. Religious traditions and beliefs provide a sense of depth and meaning at a time when we have acquired the wisdom to appreciate them. Whatever stresses we face are considerably moderated by the prayer and meditation, which are implicit in nearly all religions.

Bill Moyers's book *Healing and the Mind* looked at Eastern religions and commented that prayer and meditation are major components of Islam and Buddhism, for example, just as in Christianity and Judaism. So, all religions help in developing an awareness of a larger reality and promote an understanding that life has meaning and significance. The peace that flows from this is a good antidote for stress.

Summing Up

Times of great stress may visit you in life. Stress is one of the certitudes of living. For better or for worse, it is out there for us all. As a complex adaptive system, stress can play a positive role for you by requiring you to interact with events, adapt to them, and evolve with the changing circumstances of your life. This keeps your creative juices flowing and ensures that you are living to your fullest potential. When stressors are sufficient to overwhelm your homeostasis, it is crucial that you recognize this and take steps to cope with them. Your physical and emotional health depend on your doing this. A variety of coping techniques are available which can bolster your ability to handle stress in a positive fashion. If, in spite of all your efforts, you find that you cannot control your symptoms of stress, expert third-party help should be sought. You are entering a wonderful era in life and you deserve to enjoy it to the fullest.

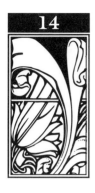

FITNESS

WE'RE TALKIN' NUTRITION
AND EXERCISE HERE, FOLKS

Were some of you hoping that I would somehow skip over these two task masters? Well, I can't. Honesty demands their inclusion in any book about menopause. Good nutrition and exercise are the major components of fitness, and being fit is one of the most worthwhile goals to achieve in midlife and beyond. In this chapter, I will make the case for healthy eating and healthy exercising.

Up until the mid-30s, many women (men too) feel that paying heed to their body's condition is merely an option. By midlife and menopause, however, fitness should be pretty near the top of your agenda if you wish to enjoy the next 30 to 40 years. As things now stand, you only get issued one body, so it is important to protect it for the great years ahead. Don't misunderstand my meaning here: Menopause is not going to make your body disintegrate like a cheap watch. Changes are going to occur, but there are steps you can take to preserve your body and diminish your chances of developing problems like heart disease, osteoporosis, and others. Did you ever see the bumper sticker that says, "If you don't take care of your body, you won't have any place to live"?

The following pages will be a discussion of good food, good eating habits, and good exercise. If you are like most, your body can use some help, but do not be intimidated. No attempt will be made to convert you to some health cult—no preaching. Incorporate these ideas and suggestions gradually into your life and lifestyle; in the long run, you will feel the benefits of having shaped up.

Nutrition

There is great cultural, ethnic, and religious diversity in our country, which makes for great diversity in the eating habits of Americans. These diverse influences are impossible to integrate into a "standard" diet, although I'll betcha some committee or other has thought about trying it. Nevertheless, there are principles of healthful nutrition that apply to all diets, regardless of origin. The fact is, most Americans do not follow these tenets regardless of race, cultural background, education, or income, so everyone can benefit from a better understanding of good nutrition.

Mountains of evidence indicate that diet has an impact on the incidence of many chronic and life-threatening diseases such as cardiovascular disease (CVD), high blood pressure, diabetes, chronic liver disease, obesity, and dental decay. There is very strong evidence that diet is involved in several forms of cancer: breast, colon, stomach, esophagus, lung.

CHANGING YOUR DIET

If your diet needs changing, some preliminaries will improve your chances of success. Doing the following will help you to get the most out of a healthful diet by getting it done right and without guilt (Cone 1993).

✦ Learn about food. Find out what foods are good for you, and what effect various foods will have on your body. Make a list of the foods you like, and a list of foods that are harmful. Many will turn up on both lists, of course. Bummer. There is plenty of literature available to provide this information, or you may already have your own library of nutrition books. One that I have found to be an excellent resource is *The New American Diet System* by Sonja and William Connor. The authors have developed a cholesterol-saturated fat index (CSI), which serves as a quick reference guide to foods that are the healthiest (Connor 1991).

✦ Be honest with yourself about your eating habits. You know what foods you like, so admit that to yourself. "Yessss. I *do* love chocolate eclairs with a large chocolate shake. A two-inch filet mignon on a canapé with foie gras, truffles and Madeira sauce is to die for. Pecan pie with two scoops of *real* ice cream is practically orgastic." Now, with that out in the open, you can go to work on making some changes that could possibly accommodate some of your greater culinary passions. While you are at it, better have a look at snacking between meals, donuts at the office, and raiding the fridge during commercials. This is not intended to give you a guilt trip, but only to urge you to identify some bad habits and recognize them for what they are. Change comes after that.

✦ Decide why you want to change. If you have gotten this far in the book, you understand that the postmenopausal years pose some serious health threats that you would like to avoid. In addition, a smaller dress size may be desirable, an admiring glance from someone important to you might be nice, and you can get rid of that lousy bathroom scale that says "one at a time please" when you stand on it.

With your new knowledge of food, your having acknowledged your own personal strengths and weaknesses about food, and now the reasons why you want to change your diet, the decision to change is at hand. It needs to be a commitment—not a resolution, but a *commitment*. It must be a deeply felt and religiouslike fervor that you will stick with for the balance of your lifetime. That balance, by the way, could prove to be a hefty one, in addition to a healthy one.

✦ Establish good eating as a daily routine. The fast pace of life in our country can make for atrocious eating habits. When you don't have time for lunch, a Big Mac, fries, and a vanilla shake may save you some time, but at great cost. You just had 1,076 calories (1,800–2,000 is about a day's worth), 49.8 grams of fat (50–60 grams for a day is recommended), 118 mg of cholesterol (less than 300 mg for a day), and 1,325 mg of sodium (less than 2,000 mg/day), and that was just lunch! (Kowalski 1990). Prepackaged and precooked foods are a lot easier to deal with than cooking from scratch. It works when time is of the essence or you are too tired to do anything else, but that doesn't make it right. So, what is a body to do? Make eating properly a higher priority on your daily agenda. Make time for it. Learn how to prepare foods more quickly, or make more time for preparation. The quickness will come with experience. Learn to be a healthy food shopper by reading the labels (more on this follows). Keep healthy snacks in the house. Fruits such as apples, oranges, apricots work. Have cold raw veggies like carrots, radishes, celery, cauliflower, green peppers in ice water. Keep unhealthy snacks (chips, nuts, dips, sweets) out of the house. If you are committed, you will learn all of this easily and your daily good-eating habits will turn out to be a no-fuss situation.

✦ Set goals you can accomplish. Keep your long-term goal in mind, of course, but don't set yourself up for failure by expecting progress that is not realistic. Failure is too hard on your body. Acknowledge your successes as you go along and *revel* in them. Dietary change is really difficult, but the long-term benefit is enormous.

FAT—AN AMERICAN EPIDEMIC

A Harris poll in January 1996 revealed that 74% of Americans weigh more than the recommended range for their corresponding height and body size. That works out to more than 200 million overweight people. That's up from 59% just 10 years ago. Americans now weigh an average of 8 pounds more than they did just 15 years ago. The Harris poll also showed that 65 million Americans (24%) are more than 20% above the recommended limit. This is the definition of obesity. Other government surveys indicate 37 million people are more than 35% overweight. Obesity costs $70 billion a year in medical treatment for its related health problems. Compared to slender people, severely overweight people run twice the risk for getting cancer, three times the risk of heart disease, and up to 40 times the risk of developing diabetes. We eat too much.

Dietary fat has long been a subject of great concern because of its close association with hardening of the arteries and, in recent years, with cancer. Fat from food is derived from any or all of the following: saturated fat, monounsaturated fat, polyunsaturated fat, and dietary cholesterol. To paraphrase Butch Cassidy and the Sundance Kid, "Who *are* these fat guys?" Let's take a look.

Saturated fat

Consumption of saturated fat is the major determining factor in raising your total blood cholesterol as well as the LDL (bad guy) cholesterol. This type of fat is usually solid at room temperature. Food sources are animal fat, dairy products made from milk, such as butter, and plant products, such as coconut oil and palm kernel oil (called *tropical oils*).

Monounsaturated fat

Monounsaturated fats (olive oil, canola oil, peanut oil) are also harmful, but less so than saturated fats. They are usually liquid at room temperature. These fats, especially olive oil, appear to be the least harmful because they have no undesirable effect on your cholesterol and may even lower slightly total cholesterol and LDL cholesterol. Like all fats, though, there are still nine calories in every gram, so weight gain can result from heavy use. There has been a lot of olive oil hoopla in recent years, after studies revealed less heart disease and breast cancer in Mediterranean cultures where their daily calories are 30%–40% from fat, and much of it from olive oil. Don't fall into the trap of believing that if olive oil is good for you, then you can start using it in great quantities on everything from pasta to salads to fish to red meat. It is still important to cut back on total fat intake.

Polyunsaturated fat

Polyunsaturated fats (corn oil, safflower oil, soybean oil, sunflower oil, cottonseed oil, fish oils) can be grouped with monounsaturated fats as less harmful than saturated fats, but with the same precautions of avoiding overuse. The oils of cold-water fish (tuna, salmon, mackerel) contain a polyunsaturated fat called *omega-3 fatty acid*. A six-year Harvard study of about 51,000 professionals (mostly dentists) showed a 25% reduction in the risk of death from coronary heart disease in those who ate one or two servings of fish per week (von Schacky 1987). There was no significant additional benefit with a higher fish intake. So, some fish is good, but more is not necessarily better. Be sure to tell your dentist.

Hydrogenated or partially hydrogenated fat

These fats and oils are also known as *trans-fatty acids*. They are merely mono- or polyunsaturated fats that have been changed to a saturated fat for longer shelf life. Margarine is a good example. A tablespoon of margarine contains up to 2 grams of saturated fat, plus another 2 grams of trans fat. That's 4 grams of "bad" fat, although it compares favorably to the 7 grams of saturated fat in butter. Trans fats raise your cholesterol just like saturated fats, but worse, they also lower your good guy HDL. Best to leave them on the shelf.

Dietary cholesterol

Dietary cholesterol is not actually a fat. It is a waxy substance called a *lipid* that is derived primarily from saturated fats, essentially all animal fat. Cholesterol is of vital importance to many normal bodily functions. It is the building block from which hormones are made. Your body makes vitamin D from cholesterol. Cholesterol forms the sheaths that protect your nerves. Your body can make all the cholesterol it needs, but the problem comes from getting too much of it from your diet. Too much of it is not good for you. The major sources of cholesterol in our diet are

+ dairy products: eggs, whole milk, cheese
+ red meat, especially if marbled with fat
+ poultry, especially if the skin is eaten
+ fish: cold-water fish like salmon, tuna, mackerel, haddock, even rainbow trout
+ shellfish: lobster, shrimp, and clams are higher in cholesterol than other seafood, but they will raise your cholesterol less than eggs and contain less saturated fat than meat and poultry. So go ahead and have that shrimp salad once in a while.
+ organ foods: liver, kidney, sweetbreads, brain (brain has 2,100 mg cholesterol per 3.5 oz serving!!)

FAT NUMBERS

The American Heart Association recommends that fat comprise no more than 30% of daily calories. Many nutritionists peg that number at 25% or less. For

85% of American women, fat comprises nearly 40% of the calories consumed each day. Fat has nine calories per gram. This works out to an allowance of around 60 grams per day for a woman consuming 1,800 calories, *if* 30% of the calories are from fat. The arithmetic is 1800 x 30% = 540 calories; 540 divided by 9 calories per gram equals 60 grams of fat per day. It is reduced to 50 grams per day if the 25% recommendation is used. A Big Mac, fries, and a vanilla shake, at 49.8 grams of fat, kind of shoots most of the day for fat, doesn't it? Heart specialist Dr. Dean Ornish restricts his patients to 10%, but these are people who have established heart disease. Ornish recommends zero animal fat for people who have already had heart attacks, *if* their heart and vascular disease is to be reversed in the specialized program he offers.

WHAT DOES FAT DO?

Dietary fat is readily converted to body fat. It is then stored in places you do not want it, like blood vessel walls and around the middle, to name but two. At nine calories per gram, fat has more than twice as many calories as carbohydrate (4.0 cal/gm) or protein (4.0 cal/gm). Very few carbohydrate calories end up as fat stores unless you are eating them with both hands. Another problem with body fat is that it is not as readily burned off for energy as carbohydrate stores, so it tends to be a bit more of a permanent fixture.

From all of the above, I think that any fair-minded person would agree that the case against fat is well made. Fat *is* needed by our bodies, but the body only needs about 15–25 grams daily to get by—not 100 grams, which is the average daily consumption in the United States. Epidemiological (broad population) studies have shown significantly lower rates of colon cancer and breast cancer in people whose fat intake is less than 20% of total daily calories. In Japan, where it is about 10%, the breast cancer death rate is less than half that of U.S. women.

"Alright already," you are probably snarling. "You've convinced me that fat is bad for me, so let's get on with it." We shall indeed press on—to carbohydrates and protein, the remaining two components of the food we eat.

CARBOHYDRATES

Carbohydrates consist of sugars, starches, and fiber. They are converted to glucose in your body and used as the primary energy source for your brain, basic body functions, and muscles. The blood glucose is either used immediately for energy or stored as *glycogen* in your liver or muscles for subsequent use. If you are "carbing out," however, the excess carbohydrate is converted to fat, and that gets stored in places where you would rather not have it, like hips and thighs.

Complex carbohydrates are the foods that should comprise at least 55%–60% of your diet. They are distinguished from sugars and sweets as foods that require enzymes to break them down for digestion. They are mostly starches and fiber such as potatoes, rice, beans, grains, plus fruits and vegetables. They contain no animal fat, and if they are not refined (as opposed to white sugar, flour, and white rice), complex carbohydrates have abundant vitamins, minerals, and fiber.

Sugar and refined starches will give you a quick energy surge from glucose, but also a quick letdown because they produce an insulin surge. Usually the insulin produced is more than you need; this results in more conversion of glucose to fat. This is why chocolate binges pack on the pounds. I wish I didn't have to tell you that. This type of "stripped" carbohydrate is low in vitamins, minerals, and fiber.

The fiber component of carbohydrates is a lot more important to your health than you may know. The average fiber intake in the American diet is only 10–20 grams per day, but 30–35 grams is the recommended amount to take advantage of fiber's benefit. Below is what friendly fiber has to offer to particular health problems.

+ *Heart disease.* Insoluble fiber in oats, oat bran, dried peas, and beans decreases your risk of coronary heart disease. Combined with a low fat diet, it helps to decrease your LDL.
+ *Diabetes.* A high fiber intake improves blood sugar control because it is more slowly absorbed from your intestine and more slowly metabolized. This helps protect against diabetes and improves control in those who are already diabetic.
+ *Cancer.* High fiber intake decreases the risk of colon cancer and may decrease the risk of many other cancers by up to one-third.
+ *Intestinal problems.* High fiber intake decreases constipation and reduces the risk of diverticulitis. Diverticula are little pouches opening out from the colon that can become inflamed and infected. They cause pain and may rupture to produce an abdominal or pelvic abscess.
+ *Weight control.* High fiber foods are low in fat and calories. They are slowly digested, which keeps you from getting hungry as soon. They also decrease starch absorption, which reduces the calories you take aboard.

While fiber intake needs to be 30–35 grams per day, it should not exceed that amount because it will decrease the amount of calcium and vitamins you can absorb. In addition, if you increase from your usual 10 grams to 35 too quickly, it can cause problems with bloating and gas. So do it, but at a measured pace.

PROTEIN

Protein is also an energy source, although carbohydrates and fat are a more accessible supply. Protein is utilized as a basic building material for your bone, muscles, blood, skin, nails, and hair. The production of hormones, antibodies, and enzymes requires protein. Proteins are composed of chains of amino acids. Your body utilizes 22 amino acids to supply all of its needs. It can make 14 of them, but the other 8 must come from food sources. These outsiders are referred to as *essential amino acids*. Meat and dairy products can supply these essential eight, but fruit and vegetables cannot. Nutritionists recommend that we eat 0.42 grams of protein per pound of body weight per day (Ojeda 1995). That works out to 55 grams if you weigh 130 pounds. Most Americans eat much more than that, and we don't need it. The excess gets stored as, you guessed it, fat.

HEALTHFUL FOOD SELECTION AND PREPARATION

Now we will cover what is good for you, and how you can keep it that way. In 1992, the United States Department of Agriculture (USDA) revised the famous 1956 "basic four" food groups: meat, dairy products, grains, fruits and

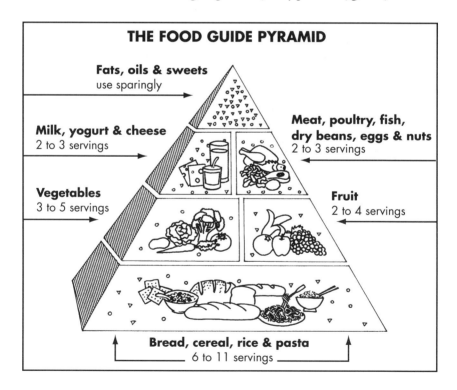

THE FOOD GUIDE PYRAMID

Fats, oils & sweets
use sparingly

Milk, yogurt & cheese
2 to 3 servings

Meat, poultry, fish,
dry beans, eggs & nuts
2 to 3 servings

Vegetables
3 to 5 servings

Fruit
2 to 4 servings

Bread, cereal, rice & pasta
6 to 11 servings

vegetables. The revision is called the *food pyramid* (see Figure 14-1). It is the result of current scientific thought about food and food's relationship to health. The foundation of the pyramid comprises the foods we should emphasize the most: complex carbohydrates consisting of bread, cereal, rice, and pasta (6–11 servings per day). These foods should be 55%–60% of our diet. The next level up is smaller: fruits (2–4 servings/day) and vegetables (3–5 servings/day). Continuing upward, the next level is two groups of proteins and is smaller still: the milk, yogurt, cheese group (2–3 servings/day) and the meat, poultry, fish, dry beans, eggs, and nuts group (2–3 servings/day). Finally, the top of the pyramid consists of the fats, oils, and sweets group, with the admonition to use sparingly.

The food pyramid should be regarded as a guideline for designing your new diet. It should help you decide what proportions of the various foods you should include on a daily basis. You don't have to eat *all* those servings every day, thank heavens—the maximum adds up to no less than 26 servings! You do that and you might end up *looking* like a pyramid! The real value of the pyramid is that it emphasizes fiber and carbohydrate as the foundation of your daily diet, rather than meat, poultry, and fish as in the past.

The American Heart Association makes the concept of "proportions" a little clearer. Table 14-1 illustrates their plan for a healthy diet.

Space doesn't permit listing examples of fat, carbohydrate, and protein foods. I'll leave that to your nutrition library. *Serving* is the word that bothers me when I read about foods. How much are they talking about when they say "a serving" of something? They always seem to leave it to your imagination. Is it a teaspoonful or a shovelful? Table 14-2 summarizes the serving plan recommended by the American Heart Institute as well as the National Academy of Sciences.

Table 14-1

RECOMMENDED DAILY FOOD PROPORTIONS

Type of food	Amount
Total fat	Less than 30% of daily calories
Saturated fat	Less than 10%
Unsaturated fat	Less than 10%
Carbohydrates (mostly complex)	More than 50% of daily calories
Protein	About 20%–25% of daily calories
Cholesterol	Less than 300 mg
Sodium	Less than 3 g

Source: Adapted from American Heart Association

Table 14-2

SERVING SIZES FOR VARIOUS FOODS

Type of food and daily amount	Serving size
Fats (less than 5–8 servings)	
Margarine or vegetable oil	1 teaspoon
Diet margarine	2 teaspoons
Peanut butter or mayonnaise	2 teaspoons
Seeds or nuts	1 teaspoon
Salad dressing	1 tablespoon
Olives	10 small or 5 large
Avocado	⅛ of a whole
Carbohydrates	
Fruits and vegetables (minimum 5 servings)	
Fruit, fresh	1 medium
Fruit, canned, cooked, chopped	½ cup
Fruit juice	¾ cup
Vegetables	½ cup
Breads, cereals, starchy vegetables (6 or more servings)	
Bread	1 slice
Cereal, flake	1 cup
Cereal, hot, low fat	½ cup
Cereal, nugget or bud-type	¼ cup
Rice or pasta, not made with egg yolks	1 cup
Starchy vegetables (corn, peas, potatoes, yams, sweet potatoes, lima beans)	½ cup
Soup, low fat	1 cup
Protein (no more than 2 servings)	
Meat, fish, poultry, cooked	3 oz.*
Meat, fish, poultry, raw	4 oz.
Vegetables (peas, lentils, cooked beans)	1 cup
Tofu	3 oz.

Adapted from American Heart Association and National Academy of Science
*Note: 3 oz is about size of deck of cards

The serving plan in Table 14-2 provides enough food that you will not feel hungry or deprived. It does indeed cut down on our American appetite for huge amounts of meat and whole milk products. For cancer prevention, however, the total calories from fat need to be even less, at 20% or below. To do this you will need to restrict your fat to three to five servings, instead of the five to eight in this serving plan. Try cooking substitutes such as broiling, steaming, and poaching without oil. Use jellies or jams without butter or margarine on your toast or muffins. Try mustard instead of mayo on your sandwich. Get nonfat salad dressings, or use just vinegar and spices. Such a diet is difficult to follow in every aspect of your life, so you will need to allow yourself some leeway at times, especially at dinner parties and when dining out.

SHOPPING SMARTS

After you have educated yourself about food (and do not neglect your food education, because food knowledge is not intuitive), then you can start becoming a smart food shopper. Take your glasses and your calculator with you while marketing, and read the labels. The labels of most prepared foods now include a nutritional analysis of the contents. The front of the package may promise "No cholesterol," but just check out the nutritional analysis. You will find that there is indeed no cholesterol, but what about total fat content? Hmm? Another ploy is "Only 100 calories per serving," but the fine print shows that a serving wouldn't fill up a thimble. Be careful of "light" and "lite" labels. A regular hot dog has 142 calories and 13.5 grams of fat. Your calculator will show you that $13.5 \times 9 = 121.5$; 121.5 of those calories, or 85%, are from fat. If you do the same figuring for what is being promoted as the "light" hot dog, you will find that 65% of its calories still come from fat. A lot has been said about how much better 2% milk is for you, but it still has about two-thirds the fat of whole milk. If the front of the package says "Low Fat," ask yourself, lower than what? and then subject it to your new steely-eyed scrutiny.

This part of your food education should probably be acquired on a day off, when you have plenty of time to browse the aisles at the market. Don't plan any purchases; just make an inventory of foods you like that fit the criteria for being healthful. Compare different brands too. Armed with your new lists, shopping will not take any more time than before. And think of the fun you will have as you vent your righteous indignation on bad foods by contemptuously turning your back on them.

The FDA was recently mandated to revise food labeling so that you have an immediate comparison of the package contents with daily recommendations for total fat, cholesterol, saturated fat, protein, fiber, carbohydrate, and sodium. Shopping for nutritious foods is a lot simpler now.

LOW FAT FOOD PREPARATION

Cooking your nutritious and wisely selected morsels is next. You are probably thinking, "I'll be damned if I'm going to eat steamed vegetables and rice for the rest of my life!" or, "What will people think if I don't serve my standing rib roast, mashed potatoes and gravy, creamy Italian salad dressing, vegetables sautéed in butter, and pumpkin pie with whipped cream?" For most Americans, taste is spelled F-A-T, and reducing fat is synonymous with bland, blah, blech. But you will be pleasantly surprised to know that low fat foods and low fat food preparations can be utterly delicious. Some very talented people have devoted some very serious effort to come up with some very innovative ways of making healthy foods taste good. Book stores and magazines racks are awash in the new literature.

It is beyond the scope of this book to teach food preparation, as well as way beyond the expertise of this author to teach cooking—my wife, Victoria, does our cooking, and she is magic. However, Table 14-3 lists a few examples of low fat food substitutes that can aid in the process of adopting a healthier diet.

OBESITY DRUGS

The world breathlessly awaits one that works. Pharmaceutical companies all over the planet have been working to that end for decades. At this time, quite a number of drugs, which are forecast to hold promise for reducing body fat, are in the research pipeline. Some are targeted for the brain areas where the chemicals related to hunger or satiety are manufactured. Some target the intestine to prevent absorption of fat. Others target the body's metabolism to speed up the burning of fat.

Two drugs that have been in common use are *fenfluramine* (Pondimin) and *phentermine* (Fastin, Banobese, Zantryl, Adipez). They were used together under the nickname "fen-phen." Phentermine is basically a stimulant which suppresses appetite and speeds up metabolism. Fenfluramine also works as an appetite suppressant by increasing the neurotransmitter brain chemical called *serotonin*. Serotonin is one of your brain's "feel good" chemicals. Higher levels reduce your feeling of hunger, and improve your mood. One three-and-a-half year study of fen-phen in people more than 50% above ideal body weight showed a 16% (25+ pounds) loss. Researchers of this study from the University of Rochester School of Medicine found that within five months of discontinu-

Table 14-3
LOW FAT FOOD SUBSTITUTES

Recipe calls for:	Substitution:
1 whole egg	2 egg whites
1 egg yolk	1 oz. Egg Beaters
Cream	Evaporated skim milk
Whole milk	Nonfat milk
Butter	Corn oil or soft margarine
Cooking oil for frying	Pam cooking spray
Buttered popcorn	Molly McButter
Sour cream	Nonfat yogurt, plain

ing fen-phen, most people had regained almost all of their original weight. The problem? The pill takers had not learned a new dietary lifestyle.

In April 1996, the FDA approved a drug called Redux (*dexfenfluramine*). This is a chemical isomer of fenfluramine, and it works much the same way by raising serotonin levels. In addition, dexfenfluramine use resulted in improved lipid levels (usually abnormally high in overweight people) and improved glucose metabolism, which is an advantage in diabetics. The FDA strongly recommended that this drug be used *only* for people who were 30%–35% overweight. Unfortunately, this admonition was not strictly observed, and "pill mills" opened by the hundreds all over the country.

Other long-term studies with fen-phen showed that over a three-year period, an average of 14–18 pounds was lost. The numbers were similar with dexfenfluramine. A serious concern for people who used fenfluramine and dexfenfluramine is the rare but potentially fatal development of pulmonary hypertension. This is a condition in which the blood vessels in your lungs become sufficiently damaged to cause heart failure and death. About half those who develop pulmonary hypertension do not survive it. An August 1996 article in the *New England Journal of Medicine* stated that the risk for this complication was 23 times higher with use of fenfluramine. It is estimated that it will occur in 23 to 46 of every 1 million users (Abenhaim 1996). In 1997 it was found that 32% of 291 people taking fenfluramine or dexfenfluramine had developed leaky heart valves. Earlier research found brain damage in laboratory animals given these drugs, but this has not been found in humans. Because of these risks, both drugs were withdrawn from the market in September 1997.

Another serotonin targeting drug called *sibutramine* is also being looked at; but it is not yet on the market. Its brand name will be Meridia.

Several genes have been discovered in humans that control obesity. Not surprisingly, one of these obesity genes has been named OB. The OB gene produces a hormone called *leptin*, which attaches to receptor sites in your brain. From those sites leptin influences how much fat your body stores. Obesity results from either inadequate amounts of leptin or brain cell receptor sites that are insensitive to leptin. Work is in progress to improve both of these parameters of fat storage control. This would be an exciting advance if it is worked out.

Still another new approach to controlling obesity involves *neuropeptide Y*, a brain chemical that in laboratory animals has been found to be a powerful stimulator of the urge to eat. Nicknamed "NPY," this chemical attaches to brain receptor sites. Research is now under way to design drugs that will prevent NPY from occupying the receptor sites, thus turning off the desire to eat.

A new drug, Xenical, that inhibits absorption of fat from the intestines is being used in Europe. Its problem is that it produces ferocious fatty diarrhea.

Users find themselves planning their day around where the nearest toilet is located.

With fenfluramine and dexfenfluramine gone, a push is under way for what is being called herbal fen-phen, a mixture that combines Saint-John's-wort from a plant source and ephedra, a Chinese herb. Saint-John's-wort enhances serotonin levels similar to fenfluramine's effect, and ephedra acts as a stimulant like phentermine. As yet there are no data to support the safety or effectiveness of this combination. Ephedra overdoses have been reported to result in states of severe agitation.

Most of these new antiobesity drugs are unlikely to result in more than a 5%–10% reduction of body weight because no long-term studies exist as to their ultimate safety. As a result, they will likely be approved for short-term use only—perhaps six months to a year. They will primarily be for those who are more than 35% overweight. Still, if short-term safety and effectiveness can be established, these new drugs can represent a reasonable jump start for people who intend to lose weight. The benefits will probably turn out to be appreciably less than becoming committed to healthful dietary lifestyle changes. Nevertheless, a good start in losing weight can be very beneficial to successfully making those changes.

Exercise

Less than one quarter of Americans engage in adequate exercise. Our culture has tended to believe that as we get older it is time to "take it easy," "slow down," "kick back" and that we need less exercise. The opposite is true. Being a couch potato is very dangerous to your health. A very large number of studies exist which demonstrate unequivocally that regular exercise dramatically slows the aging process. Indeed, exercise can be shown to actually *reverse* biological aging. Fortunately, the number of people getting regular exercise is increasing rather than decreasing. The American public has been much better advised and informed about the benefits of exercise since the early 1980s. That's fine, but still not enough people have taken up regular exercise as part of their lifestyle.

"WHY EXERCISE?"

Well, it will make you live longer, and the quality of your life will be ever so much better. You will feel better and look better and be in a better mood. It helps control hot flashes. Exercise will lower your LDL and raise your HDL cholesterol carriers, both of which are good for our team. One study showed that exercise reduced the chances of dying from *any* cause by 44% over those leading a sedentary existence (Blair 1989). It helps prevent osteoporosis. Some think it even improves your skin. Women who exercise tend to have better sex lives. And let us not forget that exercise burns calories. Exercise will improve your strength, balance, and coordination and promote an overall feeling of physical competence. This will make you feel and look younger. It even improves the functioning of your brain. A study at Harvard University's School of Public Health showed that athletes have 50% less breast cancer and 60% less cancer of the uterus, cervix, ovaries, and vagina than nonathletes. No matter whether you are in your 40s or 60s or beyond, it is not too late to incorporate exercise into your life and benefit from it. The large variety of programs available will accommodate any age, any body type, and nearly any health status. The benefits are so obvious that the decision to exercise is really a no-brainer. I'll bet you can hardly wait to get started.

GOALS AND HOW TO GET THERE

Regarding exercise, some is better than none, and more is better than some; but exactly how much is needed depends on your personal goals. Now that you are convinced and committed, decide what your fitness goals are from the listing of the most commonly stated objectives in Table 14-4.

General fitness is a broad term that includes all of these listed goals, but for most of you, the main goals turn out to be cardiovascular fitness and weight control. There is not a sole exercise program that will improve all of the fitness components simultaneously, but one can be designed for you using a variety of exercise forms, if that is your wish. If you are over 45, talk to your doctor about exercise before you start, so you will not aggravate any existing health problems. It is a good idea to have an electrocardiogram (perhaps a treadmill EKG for postmenopausal women), plus a cholesterol panel at the beginning, for a baseline.

If your goal is to minimize your risk for developing several chronic diseases such as diabetes and heart disease, lower your blood pressure, sleep better, lower your cholesterol, and improve your general sense of wellness, then current opinion is that you need to accumulate about 30 minutes of better than average physical activity each day.

Opinion seems to be changing about how much and how hard you need to exercise to become fit. The exercise formula promoted by scientific study in the mid-1980s was: 30–60 continuous minutes of light to moderate exercise, 3–5 times/week. All of it needed to be at an activity level that would keep your pulse at 50%–75% of a *target heart rate zone* during the exercise (some experts say 60%–80%). You can

Table 14-4
FITNESS GOALS
Cardiovascular fitness
Weight control
Muscular strength
Improved flexibility
Coordination and balance
Osteoporosis prevention
Better brain functioning
All of the above

Table 14-5
TARGET HEART RATE ZONE

Age	Target heart rate at 50%–75% maximum heart rate	Average maximum heart rate = 100%
20	100–150	200
25	98–146	195
30	95–142	190
35	93–138	185
40	90–135	180
45	88–131	175
50	85–127	170
55	83–123	165
60	80–120	160
65	78–116	155
70	75–113	150

Adapted from the American Heart Association

calculate your target heart rate zone by subtracting your age from 220 and multiplying by 50%–75%. Table 14-5 adapted from the American Heart Association (AHA) does it for you. Studies by AHA and Harvard showed that women who followed this formula had a 50% decline in deaths from all causes.

In 1995, the Centers for Disease Control and Prevention together with the American College of Sports Medicine put a new twist on the formula. Their studies indicated that moderate fitness can be achieved by accumulating 30 minutes of moderate-intensity activity at least six days per week, but preferably every day. They also found that it isn't necessary for the exercise to be continuous. It can be in 8–10 minute segments as long as the total adds up to 30 minutes and you burn about 200 calories per day in whatever activity is employed. The intensity should be comparable to brisk walking, which burns four to seven calories per minute. Activities can include calisthenics, conditioning exercise classes, dancing, racket sports, swimming, climbing stairs, raking leaves, and even house cleaning. This last one done at a brisk walking pace would make you something of a whirlwind around the place. Might stir up more dust than you can clean up. If your goal is to be more than moderately fit, you can step it up a notch with activities that burn more than seven calories per minute. See Table 14-6 for some suggestions and comparisons of these exercises. Both of the above fitness formulas work, so do whatever fits your schedule. The advantage of the daily-accumulation method is that you don't necessarily need a health club to achieve moderate fitness.

Table 14-6

SUGGESTED EXERCISE AND COMPARISONS

Moderate (4–7 calories/minute)	Strenuous (over 7 calories/minute)
Brisk walking, 3–4 mph	Brisk walking, uphill or carrying weights
Aerobic exercise, calisthenics	Aerobic exercise, stair step machine, ski machine
Swimming, moderate effort	Swimming, fast crawl
Cycling, under 10 mph	Cycling, over 10 mph
Racket sports, table tennis	Tennis singles, racquetball
Canoeing, 2–4 mph	Canoeing 3–5 mph
Mowing lawn, power mower	Mowing lawn, hand mower
Home care, general cleaning	Home care, moving furniture
Golf, walking	Golf does not qualify as strenuous activity
Fishing, standing/casting	Fishing in moving stream

Adapted from American Heart Association and Academy of Sports Medicine

SET YOUR GOALS AND GO FOR THEM

The following is a brief discussion of each of the fitness goals, with suggestions for activities that will be beneficial in achieving them (ACOG 1992).

Cardiovascular fitness

To attain cardiovascular fitness, exercise at a level that maintains your heart rate in the target heart rate zone for 20 to 30 minutes, at least three times per week. You can calculate your target heart rate using the formula mentioned above: $(220 - age) \times 50\%–75\%$. As your fitness improves, you will notice that you can increase the amount of exercise you are doing and still maintain your heart rate in the 50%–75% target range. Significant CV fitness will take 12 to 16 weeks.

A "cool down" period should always follow aerobic exercise. This can be easy activity such as walking around until your heart rate is back to near normal. During exercise, large amounts of blood are diverted into your muscles and skin. If you stop suddenly, the blood is rushed back into the central circulation; this may cause dizziness, nausea, or fainting. Also, do not jump into a hot shower or a hot tub or a sauna until your heart rate has slowed. The heat on your skin will cause more blood to be diverted from your central circulation to your skin. This can make your blood pressure drop too low to properly supply your heart or your brain.

Weight control

Exercise can be useful for weight loss and weight maintenance. A weight management program that combines both exercise and diet is more effective in the long term than a program based on either one alone. A particular benefit of exercise is that it seems to preferentially utilize central abdominal fat more than other sites. Since abdominal fat has a significant correlation with heart disease, this is an added benefit. So is a more slender waist line.

Weight loss from exercise is slow and results from burning up more calories than you take in. A negative calorie balance occurs. Each pound of body fat contains 3,500 kilocalories (kcal). If you burn 500 kcal per hour in moderate exercise activity, it takes 7 such sessions to lose a pound of body weight. This assumes your dietary intake stays the same. Yep, that's slow. If you are also on a weight losing diet, then weight loss will occur at a faster rate. A precaution here, is that you should not diet severely while on an exercise program, since you do need energy to sustain the increased physical activity. Let us not forget, if this is a permanent change in your way of living, the weight is gone for good, so you can afford to be patient.

The best formula for weight loss with exercise is to include 30–60 minutes of exercise, 5 or 6 days each week at the 50%–75% target range for heart rate. A myth has been circulating in the fitness industry for nearly a decade that more fat is burned by slower physical activity than with vigorous activity. It was the result of a misinterpretation of research that showed a higher percentage of fat than carbohydrate is burned with less intense activity, and a higher percentage of carbohydrate than fat is burned with vigorous activity. Therefore slow down and lose fat, right? Wrong, folks. The facts are that your body utilizes its two main fuel sources, carbohydrate and fat, in any level of activity. With intense activity, your body calls on easy-to-metabolize carbohydrates more than harder-to-burn fat, but fat is not ignored. Fat gets burned too. The bottom line is that you burn far more fat in an hour of intense activity than in an hour of less intense activity. Another way of putting it is that for a 150-pound person to burn 300 calories by walking, it takes 69 minutes at 3 mph, 52 minutes at 4 mph, and 27 minutes at 5 mph. So get out there and start huffing and puffing at a rate that works for you.

Muscle is the most metabolically active tissue in your body, so it is important to retain muscle mass in a weight management program. The more muscle you have, the more calories you burn. In the early stages of an exercise program, you will be building muscle, which weighs twice as much as fat per unit of volume. This means you could be losing fat without a net loss in weight, but just notice how your clothes fit more loosely. After your muscles are strengthened, your continued fat loss will reflect itself in more rapid body weight loss.

Muscle strength

For a muscle to be strengthened, it must be contracted against resistance. Currently popular exercise programs tend to emphasize the lower body (aerobic dancing, steps classes, brisk walking, jogging). If you wish to improve arm strength and your upper body, it will require a different set of exercises. Free weight lifting, fitness machines, or handheld weights while you are doing aerobics can fill the bill. Swimming is also very good for upper body strengthening. Weight training machines and weight lifting programs generally do not contribute significantly to cardiovascular fitness, although a 1989 study by Franklin did report that upper body training programs could be designed for aerobic benefit.

Flexibility

Stiffening up with the passage of years can be avoided by a systematic stretching program. Most aerobic programs start with a "warm up" or stretching routine. Some experts disagree on whether stretching is most beneficial before or after exercise; most seem to favor stretching before *and* after. Self-directed stretching commonly causes muscle, ligament, and joint injuries, so get some expert advice first.

Coordination and balance

Lack of coordination and balance results in many falls and mishaps for postmenopausal women. Exercise involving repetitive tasks is particularly helpful in improving coordination and balance. Any activity done repeatedly over a period of time will develop neuromuscular pathways to the point that the activity becomes reflex in nature. Good examples are typing or playing the piano. As you become better trained, your ability to perform accurately improves. Exercise works the same way to make you more competent in using your body, and the result is fewer injuries. With competence comes confidence, and you will look fit because you stand straighter, walk with grace, and have a confident step.

Osteoporosis prevention

Higher bone densities are seen in active women than in sedentary women. Fitness exercises such as aerobics or muscle strengthening will improve bone density by placing stress on your bones. Swimming, while it is good aerobic exercise, does not put much stress on bone, and little change is seen. Same for casual walking, although brisk walking is quite helpful. The evidence to date is that exercise, like calcium and estrogen, is needed on a continual basis to prevent osteoporosis.

Better brain functioning

This doesn't top the list for most because it is relatively new information. Brain research is not new, but only recent studies have shown a close relationship between body movement and learning. Researchers have found that your brain becomes conditioned by exercise in much the same way as muscles, the heart, and bone. Brain cells are helped by increased blood flow during exercise. In addition, growth of cells is facilitated by a greater supply of natural substances called *neurotrophins*. It was found that everyone's capacity to process new, and remember old, information is enhanced by aerobic exercise. This is true for children as well as for adults at any age. It has also been found that if the aerobic exercise involves complex and coordinated movements, such as aerobic dancing, more new brain pathways are created than by simpler activities like aerobic walking. Other examples of complex activities include swimming, tennis, squash, racquetball, and handball. Simpler forms of exercise (gardening, raking leaves, stair climbing) work too, but not quite as well. All of these activities make the brain better able to process information of all kinds. Some of the research was done on young students, who showed improved academic results. Most of it involved the elderly who had already experienced a slowdown in brain functioning. It is concluded that people in midlife can avert the typical brain drain of aging if exercise becomes part of their lifestyle.

Two studies published in the *Journal of the American Medical Association* in April 1995, showed that walking at 4 to 5 miles per hour, 5 times per week prolonged life. In a 5-year exercise study of people over 60, the death rate from *any* cause was 44% lower than in sedentary and unfit people. Reaction time, which starts slowing in the mid-30s, is not so much related to aging as it is to fitness. All this suggests that not only will exercise help you to remember where you put the blasted car keys, but also you will be a safer driver (improved gas pedal to brake pedal time) when you finally do get it started.

SUGGESTED ACTIVITIES FOR ACCOMPLISHING YOUR GOALS

Cardiovascular fitness

Jogging or walking are the most frequently utilized aerobic exercises. Jogging 20 to 30 minutes or brisk walking 45 to 60 minutes, 3 to 5 times per week will result in cardiovascular fitness for anyone. Same for accumulating 30 minutes daily of any moderate-intensity activity in 8- to 10-minute segments. Jogging is very hard on joint surfaces and ligaments, so caution is necessary. For osteoporotic women, jogging can cause fractures.

Swimming is great for upper and lower body fitness. Since it is low impact, it is well suited for women with osteoporosis in preventing fractures, but it has no beneficial effect on bone density. Some women may be interested in being rated in their swimming competence and compared to others of similar age.

If competitive swimming appeals to you, contact

US Masters Swimming
Two Peter Avenue
Rutland, MA 01543

Bicycling, rowing, and cross country skiing are all effective aerobic activities but require certain geographic requirements to be practical. Not too many women in Florida do cross country skiing on a regular basis, nor do women in Minnesota row much when the lakes are frozen. But with all the advertising on TV, I feel certain it has not escaped your notice that indoor machines are available to provide these activities.

Circuit training has become popular in many areas. It involves running, jumping, climbing, pulling, and pushing exercises. The sequential combination of these activities provides both aerobic fitness and muscle strengthening, plus relief from the boredom of a single activity. You may find this type of training through your local recreation department or a health club.

Muscle strength and tone

A muscle must have resistance to its action in order to improve its strength or size. Methods to accomplish this include lifting weights, isometric exercise, elastic resistance, body weight resistance such as push ups, or weight training machines. Utilize a trained instructor not only to avoid injury, but also to be sure your program is exercising the muscles you wish to strengthen. Of course, we're not talking about turning you into a middle linebacker, but a flatter tummy, smaller thighs, a trimmer fanny, and a firmer upper body might be nice.

PREVENTION OF INJURY

Injury avoidance revolves around using your common sense: start any new program slow and easy, acquire the proper footwear or gear, avoid high impact exercise, maintain a high hydration level while exercising, and remain alert to any signs that your body is not tolerating the exercise. A well-designed fitness program should not result in any pain for you. "No pain, no gain" is hog wash. Muscle pain means either you are exceeding your aerobic capacity or you have injured yourself. Warning signs of overexertion are

+ sudden sharp pain
+ excessive fatigue
+ difficulty breathing, not just heavy breathing
+ feeling faint or dizzy
+ nausea or vomiting
+ irregular heart beat
+ excessive muscle soreness
+ persistent lethargy after exercise

Summing Up

I would like to reiterate my earlier statement that good nutrition and exercise are the major components of fitness. Each of them is important individually, but when combined as part of your lifestyle they have potent influences on wellness. Achieving good nutrition requires commitment to a balanced diet, knowledge of food, careful food shopping, and thoughtful food preparation. Once you have these ducks all in a row, you are absolutely in charge of this aspect of maintaining a healthy body. Exercise programs for women at midlife serve many purposes including cardiovascular fitness, strength, weight control, flexibility, coordination and balance, improved bone density, and improved brain function. When you initiate your program, decide in advance what you want out of it, and tailor it to those goals. Don't be intimidated by the floor-to-ceiling mirrors, or the Spandex-clad slender young women at the health club. Their reason for being there is probably a great deal different than yours. Just keep your goal before you all the time: fitness and health to enjoy the next third of life.

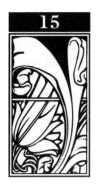

15

MENOPAUSE FROM OTHER CAUSES

Surgical menopause, chemical menopause, radiation-induced menopause, and premature menopause are all associated with special problems for women, since they generally happen at a younger age than does natural menopause. These young women often do not have peers who are menopausal. They feel singled out by bad luck and by having no friends who can relate to their problem. Most are unprepared for the health situation that has resulted in their early menopause, and their partners are unprepared as well. The health problem itself (cancer, hemorrhage, serious infection, pain) will usually have been of such primacy in a woman's mind that menopause resulting from treatment was not given serious consideration. Yet it deserves attention, because the menopausal symptoms are sudden in appearance and usually experienced with much more exaggerated symptoms than those of natural menopause. Finally, long-term menopausal threats, such as heart disease and osteoporosis, may never even make it to the surface of conscious thought for young women.

For those of you who may be faced with such problems, the following will help you organize your thinking through the complex issues involved. This chapter will aid you in making the decisions necessary for treatment of your health problem, as well as in managing your menopause.

Hysterectomy

One-third of American women will have had a hysterectomy by age 60 (Carlson 1993). It is the second most common major female operation.

Cesarean section ranks first. The National Center for Health Statistics reports that 600,000 hysterectomies are performed each year with an annual cost to the health care system of $5 billion. Regional differences exist, with many more hysterectomies done in the southern United States than in the North. International data show that countries with government controlled health care systems have fewer hysterectomies than countries like ours with private health care. Individual differences in beliefs about hysterectomy exist not only among physicians, but among patients as well. The study cited above documented that individual physicians vary in their opinions as to what constitutes valid indications for recommending the operation. All this suggests that women to whom this surgery is recommended should inform themselves thoroughly about the operation, its consequences, risks, and expected benefit. New technologies have reduced the number of hysterectomies by 20%. These newer modalities constitute valid alternatives in many instances. So, learn all you can about hysterectomy and alternatives, because medical practice in dealing with indications for this surgery is changing rapidly.

SOME MEDICAL LINGO

The operation can be done either with an abdominal incision requiring four to five days hospitalization or through the vagina with a one- to two-day hospital stay. Vaginal hysterectomies are also being done with an abdominal laparoscope. It is called *laparoscopically assisted vaginal hysterectomy* (LAVH). This technique involves several small abdominal incisions (usually four) through which the laparoscope (tube to look through) and other instruments are inserted to do the surgery. When the uterus has been detached, it is removed through the vagina. The advantages of LAVH are that the surgeon has better visibility than with a vaginal operation, and recovery is less painful than with a large abdominal incision.

The terms your doctor might use in describing the various types of operation are

✦ *total hysterectomy:* removal of the entire uterus including the cervix. Ovaries and fallopian tubes are not removed
✦ *subtotal* or *partial hysterectomy:* the cervix is left in place (also called supracervical). Ovaries are not removed. Not a very common operation in the past 40 years, since the cervix remains at risk for cancer when left in place. Recently, it is being used more frequently again in women at low risk for cervical cancer
✦ *total abdominal hysterectomy with bilateral salpingo-oophorectomy:* removal of the entire uterus, both tubes and both ovaries through an abdominal incision

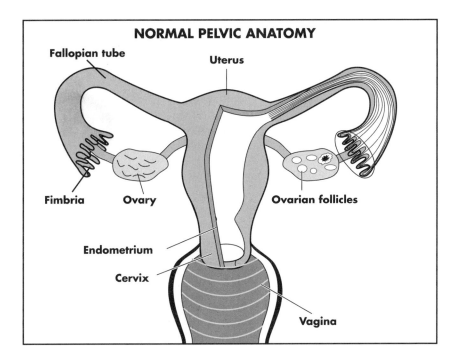

NORMAL PELVIC ANATOMY

Fallopian tube

Uterus

Fimbria   Ovary

Ovarian follicles

Endometrium

Cervix

Vagina

✦ *vaginal hysterectomy:* entire uterus is removed through your vagina, with no abdominal incision

✦ *laparoscopically-assisted vaginal hysterectomy (LAVH):* entire uterus removed through your vagina, but much of the surgery is done abdominally with video-camera viewing via the laparoscope. The laparoscope and other surgical instruments are inserted through four small abdominal incisions

✦ *salpingectomy:* removal of a fallopian tube

✦ *oophorectomy:* removal of an ovary (also called ovariectomy). It is important to know that immediate menopause results only if *both* ovaries are surgically removed

Review Figure 15-1, which is a drawing of normal pelvic anatomy. Then look over Figure 15-2, which illustrates in dark outline the anatomic structures removed in various pelvic operations.

WHY GET ONE?

Considerable thought and study has been given to formalizing and prioritizing the indications for hysterectomy. They generally fall into two categories: elective and nonelective. The firm and undisputed indications for a *nonelective* hysterectomy include

◆ invasive cancer of the cervix or endometrium (responsible for about 11% of hysterectomies)
◆ life threatening hemorrhage
◆ uncontrollable and/or life threatening infection
◆ uterine obstruction of the urinary tract or bowel

As you can see, these indications are all urgent or emergency situations in which your interests are not well served by delay.

Elective indications are less urgent and allow for advance planning. These include

◆ uterine fibroids
◆ persistent abnormal bleeding

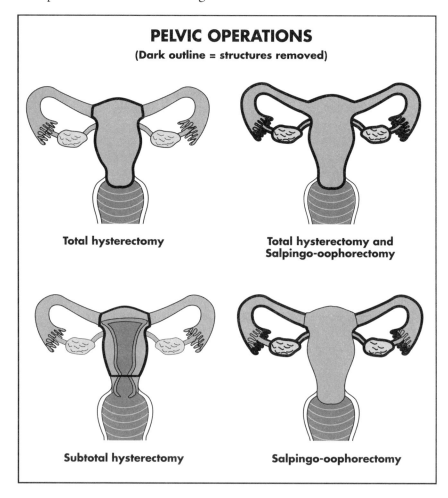

PELVIC OPERATIONS
(Dark outline = structures removed)

Total hysterectomy

Total hysterectomy and Salpingo-oophorectomy

Subtotal hysterectomy

Salpingo-oophorectomy

- ✦ endometriosis
- ✦ precancerous conditions of the uterus
- ✦ prolapse of the uterus
- ✦ chronic pelvic pain

Each of these elective indications will be discussed below.

Fibroids

Fibroids are benign (noncancerous) muscle tumors that have developed in or on the wall of the uterus. Rarely, a malignancy called *leiomyosarcoma* develops; it resembles a fibroid, but fibroids themselves are never malignant. A fibroid may also be called a *myoma*. They grow slowly but can attain the size of your head sometimes. They may take form as a single tumor but more often are multiple. Most of the time, fibroids produce no symptoms, and you might never be aware of their presence until they are felt by your doctor during a pelvic examination. The bad news is that the engine of fibroid growth is your own estrogen. The good news is that menopausal reduction of estrogen slows or stops the growth. In time they usually shrink in postmenopausal women. As many as 30% of women over age 40 have fibroids. They are more common in African-American women than women of other races. Fibroids account for 33% of all hysterectomies.

When large enough, fibroids cause a feeling of weight in the pelvis somewhat akin to a bearing down sensation. Back pain may also be experienced. When fibroids protrude into the cavity of the uterus, chronic bleeding may occur, often profuse or persistent enough to cause anemia. Occasionally, fibroids may distort the uterus sufficiently to prevent a successful pregnancy. A single large fibroid may cause pain or obstruction by exerting pressure against the bladder, a ureter (tube from the kidney to the bladder), or the intestine. Figure 15-3 is an illustration of a uterus with multiple fibroids in various locations. When a fibroid is on the outside surface of the uterus beneath its serous covering, it is called a *subserous* fibroid. If it is contained within the wall of the uterus, it is *intramural*. If it protrudes into the inner cavity beneath the mucous lining tissue, it is a *submucous* fibroid. Submucous fibroids are the ones that bleed and bleed and bleed. In 80% of women, fibroids do not produce any symptoms and require no treatment. Removal of the uterus removes fibroids, but alternative strategies may also be employed in specific situations to avoid a hysterectomy.

- ✦ *Myomectomy.* This is an operation for removal of only the fibroid or fibroids, leaving the uterus in place. This is done by an open abdominal operation if the fibroids are large, but small fibroids can also be removed with a laparoscopic operation. This surgery involves three or four Band-Aid size incisions in the abdomen, through which a

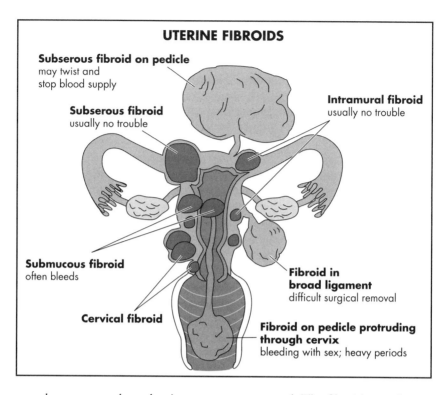

UTERINE FIBROIDS

Subserous fibroid on pedicle
may twist and
stop blood supply

Subserous fibroid
usually no trouble

Intramural fibroid
usually no trouble

Submucous fibroid
often bleeds

Cervical fibroid

Fibroid in broad ligament
difficult surgical removal

Fibroid on pedicle protruding through cervix
bleeding with sex; heavy periods

laparoscope plus other instruments are passed. The fibroids can then be destroyed by laser vaporization or by detaching them from the uterus and removing them piecemeal through the laparoscope. For fibroids protruding into the cavity of the uterus, a vaginal operation can be performed through a resectascope. This is a multichanneled instrument with fiberoptic lighting, which is passed through the cervix. A special solution is used to expand the uterine cavity for visibility, and the operative instruments are passed through the channels. Fibroids are removed by cutting them away with a loop cautery instrument. They can also be vaporized with a laser instrument called a Vapor Trode.

✦ *Laparoscopic myolysis.* This is an outpatient operation performed through a laparoscope. Electrocautery needles are placed into the fibroid and the blood supply is destroyed. This causes the fibroid to permanently shrink in size by about 50%. Since it is a relatively recent operation, it is not known what effect myolysis will have on subsequent pregnancies. If pregnancy is not on your plate for the future, this is a good way to get rid of small symptomatic fibroids without a hysterectomy.

- ✦ *Fibroid embolization.* In 1995, French physician Dr. J. H. Ravina and coworkers reported their success in destroying fibroids by passing small particles through the arteries that supply blood to the uterus. The particles plugged up the blood vessels supplying the fibroids, but the uterus was left intact. The operation is done under X-ray guidance and involves no surgery. There is a great deal of postoperative pain as the fibroids die and a profuse vaginal discharge ensues. No one knows whether successful pregnancy is possible following embolization, but it is certainly an attractive option for women with symptomatic fibroids who prefer not to have surgery.
- ✦ *Nonsurgical treatments.* Lupron-Depot shots or Synarel nasal spray are used to shrink fibroids. In most cases, the fibroid will grow again after treatment. Lupron-Depot and Synarel are used mainly as a preoperative technique to shrink the fibroids, making the surgery safer and easier. Lupron-Depot can often decrease the size sufficiently to make a vaginal, rather than an abdominal, hysterectomy possible. Recovery from the vaginal operation is quicker and less painful. Lupron-Depot is given in two or three monthly injections, but at $250 per shot, it is expensive. Check your insurance to be sure it is covered. Long-term use of these drugs, called *GnRH agonists*, has not been advocated because they stop production of your estrogen and progesterone, resulting in menopausal symptoms plus the risk of osteoporosis and CVD. This can be controlled, however, by adding back estrogen and progesterone in the same low doses used in HRT. You are menopause-protected, and the add-back therapy does not cause fibroids to regrow. GnRH agonists must be stopped after six months. If definitive surgery has not been carried out by that time, the fibroids will regrow, and you are back to square one.
- ✦ *Watch and wait.* This is a reasonable alternative for women who are close to menopause and in whom an urgent situation does not exist. Monitoring is easily carried out by periodic pelvic examinations or by pelvic ultrasound to measure the size of the fibroids. Hormone replacement is still possible for postmenopausal women with fibroids, since the dosage of estrogen in HRT is so small that fibroids are not usually adversely affected.

Abnormal and persistent bleeding

This problem accounts for about 20% of all hysterectomies. Polyps inside the uterus are a very common cause. These are small pieces of tissue that are attached to the endometrium by a stalk. Polyps are not shed by a menstrual period, so they hang on and bleed in a persistent trickle. Endometrial and cervical cancers have a similar pattern of bleeding.

Another common source of abnormal bleeding is from failure to ovulate regularly, as seen in perimenopausal women. Without ovulation, inadequate amounts of progesterone result in a thickened endometrium that is not shed as readily as usual. The common term for this is *dysfunctional uterine bleeding*, or DUB. This pattern of bleeding may be too much, too often, or both.

Evaluation for abnormal bleeding is typically done in the office by endometrial biopsy and/or by inserting a hysteroscope into the uterus through the cervix for a direct look and more accurately directed biopsies. If polyps are seen, they can usually be removed through the hysteroscope. If the biopsy discloses DUB, hormone treatment usually handles it, using low dose birth control pills, medroxyprogesterone acetate (Provera), or GnRH agonists such as Lupron-Depot or Synarel. If a cancer is found, hysterectomy is appropriate treatment.

A more recent method for dealing with abnormal bleeding from benign causes is *endometrial ablation*. This technique employs either laser vaporization or electrocoagulation with a heated roller-ball or roller-cylinder probe to destroy the uterine lining. It is an operating room procedure which is performed through a hysteroscope. To date, most of the experience is with postmenopausal women, especially those who may be poor candidates for a hysterectomy because of health problems. It is difficult to remove every single bit of endometrium with ablation techniques. The postoperative course may be fraught with continued bleeding, although it is much reduced or stopped in 80%–90% of cases. Because of the small endometrial fragments left behind after endometrial ablation, the risk of endometrial cancer persists just as in any other woman. If estrogen replacement is used, progestin must also be added.

Pelvic endometriosis

This condition accounts for 18% of hysterectomies. It is caused by endometrial cells becoming located in areas other than just the lining of the uterus. The most common sites for these errant cells are pelvic structures such as the ovaries, fallopian tubes, surface of the uterus, bladder, large intestine, lining of the pelvis, and vagina. Like the endometrial cells lining the uterus, endometriotic cells are very sensitive to female hormones and undergo the same periodic bleeding. The problem is that the bleeding causes local irritation at the nonuterine sites. This is then healed by scarring, as with any other irritation. Scarring at these various places creates adhesions and pain. Chronic pain from endometriosis is the most significant problem for perimenopausal women. In young women, involvement of the fallopian tubes is a very common source of infertility.

Surgical treatment has been total hysterectomy with removal of both ovaries to stop the hormonal stimulation of the endometriotic cells. Natural menopause usually accomplishes the same thing. Alternative treatment may involve stopping ovarian function for a few months with drugs like Lupron-Depot or Danazol. This allows the involved areas to shrink and become inactive. Birth control pills have been used for the same purpose. Laparoscopic surgery using laser vaporization and/or resection (removal) of the involved tissue has also been successful, but it is not curative. There is no permanent cure for endometriosis short of menopause or removal of the uterus and ovaries.

Precancerous conditions

If alternative treatment methods fail to control precancerous uterine conditions, a hysterectomy may be necessary. In the cervix, a condition called *high grade squamous intraepithelial lesion* (HGSIL) may become severe enough to warrant a hysterectomy. HGSIL is the term for what you may have known in the past as dysplasia or cervical intraepithelial neoplasia (CIN). HGSIL is usually treated by surgical removal of the abnormal tissue without hysterectomy. A recent method utilizes high frequency radio wave energy transmitted through a wire loop called LEEP (loop electrosurgical excision procedure). The wire loop is used to scoop away the abnormal tissue, and for many gynecologists it is the treatment of choice for HGSIL.

Precancerous endometrial hyperplasia (thickening) can be reversed by a course of progesterone therapy. Endometrial ablation is not a satisfactory method for this condition, since small fragments of endometrium are commonly left behind. These fragments can later develop into cancer.

Uterine prolapse

This refers to a sagging downward of the uterus because of loose supporting structures. Prolapse accounts for 16% of hysterectomies. The looseness occurs from stretching during childbirth and/or from loss of elasticity after menopause. Occasionally, the uterus may protrude clear outside the vagina. Vaginal hysterectomy is an appropriate and commonly used treatment. An alternative to surgery is the use in the vagina of a *pessary*, which holds the uterus in place. Lifelong Kegel exercises started after childbirth and HRT started at menopause may help to prevent prolapse.

Chronic pelvic pain

This is a devilish problem for both the woman suffering from it, and her physician who must try to relieve her of it. Pelvic pain is generally regarded as chronic when it has persisted for at least six months. Common gynecologic causes are endometriosis and scarring from pelvic infections such as sexually transmitted diseases. Chronic inflammatory bowel disease such as diverticulitis contribute to pain. A diverticulum is a pouch or pocket protruding from the large intestine. It can become inflamed and may rupture, producing a pelvic abscess. Psychological factors also play a prominent role in pelvic pain. In 1990,

Dr. R. C. Rector reported that nearly 40% of women with chronic pelvic pain had experienced childhood sexual abuse. In this situation, psychological care, not surgery, is needed.

Hysterectomy is a last ditch effort to relieve chronic pelvic pain, but it still accounts for 10% of hysterectomies. The problem is that it may not end the symptoms at all. Therefore, it is of great importance to know the *exact* source of the pain before resorting to surgery. If your gynecologist or other primary physician is unable to pinpoint the problem, your interests would be very well served by getting a psychiatric evaluation. It could save you a useless operation.

A surgical alternative to hysterectomy for pain relief is to insert a laparoscope to cut the nerve fibers that pass through ligaments behind your uterus. The Centers for Disease Control reported that this procedure was successful in 60% of patients. Laparoscopy is usually necessary to investigate pelvic conditions before resorting to hysterectomy for chronic pain anyway, so it is worth a try.

SHOULD OVARIES BE REMOVED WITH HYSTERECTOMY?

This is a difficult question to which there is no easy answer. The primary rationale for ovarian removal is prevention of cancer. Ovarian cancer is the leading cause of death from gynecologic malignancy and the fourth most frequent cause of female death from cancer in the United States. About one woman in 70 will develop ovarian cancer during her lifetime. Our ability to diagnose ovarian cancer is woefully inadequate because there are no reliable tests to detect this disease in an early stage, the only time when it counts. About 75% of malignant ovarian tumors have already spread when first detected. Physical examination and ultrasound can detect ovarian enlargement; but once an ovary has become enlarged from cancer, it has already begun to spread. It is a very discouraging disease.

Additional reasons for ovarian removal during a hysterectomy are

✦ Ovarian cancer risk factors. If you have two first-degree relatives (mother, sisters) who have had ovarian cancer, you may have a 50% chance of developing it yourself. If you have had prior malignancies such as breast, colon, rectal, or uterine cancer, your chances of ovarian cancer are increased.

✦ Limited remaining ovarian function. If you are close to menopause, you may consider the remaining productive life of your ovaries too brief to justify retaining your ovaries.

✦ Hysterectomy shortens ovarian life. A hysterectomy removes part of the blood supply to your ovaries. As many as 30% of women who retain their ovaries will be menopausal within four years because of the diminished blood supply (Loft 1993).

- Ovarian cysts. Painful and recurrent ovarian cysts occur in 10% of women who have had a hysterectomy. They are benign but do hurt, and one or both ovaries may need to be removed in a second operation.
- Severe endometriosis or premenstrual syndrome. Both of these conditions are cured by ovarian removal.

Reasons for ovarian conservation include

- Age. If there is an expectation of many remaining years for ovarian function, removal may not be advisable for you.
- Freedom from cancer is only 90% likely. During fetal life, the developing ovaries leave "rests" of ovarian cells in the abdominal lining. These cells can develop into ovarian cancer even though your ovaries have been removed.
- Regulation of hormone replacement is difficult. This problem is common to younger women in their 30s or early 40s whose estrogen requirements are higher. Estrogen replacement is not a good substitute for the way ovarian hormone production can respond to day-to-day needs.
- You are willing to take the risk. If the risks of ovarian retention are within your comfort level, you may decide to keep them. It is absolutely your call.

Most physicians recommend that you retain your ovaries if you are under age 40, encourage retention to age 45, follow the patient's preference after 45, and remove them if postmenopausal. Your decision to remove or conserve ovaries should be based on three considerations.

1. Are they still functioning, and how long can I expect that to continue?
2. How likely is it that I will need future ovarian surgery?
3. Do I have risk factors that would shorten my life if my ovaries are not removed?

So, removal of ovaries during a hysterectomy must be a carefully considered decision by women and physicians alike. It is a momentous decision which can profoundly influence your subsequent life.

RECOVERY FROM HYSTERECTOMY

Following hysterectomy, some women require months instead of weeks to fully recover. Both physical and psychological factors may play a role. Physical effects include brief episodes of menopausal symptoms even if the ovaries have been conserved. Hot flashes, depression, headaches, and palpitations can be relieved by estrogen during this time. If ovaries have been retained, the symptoms will disappear as recovery progresses; estrogen can be discontinued, generally by six weeks.

Sexual discomfort after a hysterectomy is quite common. It is usually noticed on deep penetration because this is the area where the uterus was detached from the vagina. This vaginal area is reattached to pelvic ligaments during surgery to prevent prolapse of the vagina years later. As in any area of healing, pressure is painful. After healing is completed, pain with sex will disappear, but gentleness is necessary until that has happened.

If both ovaries were removed, dramatic menopausal symptoms appear by about the second postoperative day. Hot flashes, irritability, and depression may be quite intense in premenopausal women. Sexual desire may be deeply depressed if ovaries are removed. Dr. Barbara Sherwin at McGill University has shown this to be avoidable if testosterone is added to estrogen supplements immediately after the operation. In postmenopausal women, little difference at all may be noticed.

When neither ovary is removed, hormone production continues at its normal pace. Nevertheless one-third of these women will become menopausal at an earlier age than the expected 51. Diminished blood supply is thought to be responsible, because a branch of the uterine artery that supplies the ovary is cut during a hysterectomy. The main blood supply from the ovarian artery is left intact. In general, the closer a woman is to menopause at the time of surgery, the shorter is the remaining ovarian function. For example, at age 46, function may stop in 2 to 4 years, but at age 30 it is more likely to be another 16 to 18 years.

A commonly described psychological result of hysterectomy is depression. Dr. Carlson and her colleagues in their 1993 study found no general association between hysterectomy and major depression. Their work showed that depression had actually preceded the surgery in most cases. In spite of this, many women voice feelings of sadness at the loss of their reproductive option and say that they feel less than whole. They resent tactless comments by other women who may not place the same value on this physical representation of womanhood as they do. Furthermore, some men are so turned off by a woman without a uterus that they end the relationship. This can be a further loss for a woman to contend with after surgery.

GET READY FOR IT

Much of the psychological stress pertaining to hysterectomy can be avoided by good preoperative preparation on the part of the woman who is to have the surgery. Be sure you know what operation you are having, how it is to be done, what aftereffects can be expected, what complications are possible, plus the risks and expected benefits. Your doctor should provide you with all of this information, and you should make sure that all of your questions are answered to your satisfaction. If the surgery will make you menopausal, then a complete discussion of menopause is due to you. Find out how much the operation costs, and see what your insurance covers. Know what hospital is to be used, what tests you might need, and how long you may be hospitalized. Your partner should be involved in these discussions, and any other household member should be apprised of what is being planned.

Preoperative preparation may include talking to other women who have had the operation, contact with a hysterectomy support group, a second physician's opinion, and perhaps a telephone consultation with HERS (Hysterectomy Educational Resources and Services) Foundation. This organization offers free counseling via telephone regarding hysterectomy, alternatives to hysterectomy, and strategies for dealing with postoperative effects of the operation.

Posthysterectomy psychological problems and surprises can be minimized if you are well prepared intellectually, if you have solicited social support from your family and friends, and if you have confronted the psychological issues that could arise for you. By preparing carefully and thoroughly, hysterectomy will be much less stressful for you and less confusing for those around you.

Chemotherapy and Radiation Therapy

When cancer is diagnosed, no one is prepared for the sudden and wrenching changes that will intrude upon them. Survival takes precedence over nearly all else. For women, cancer treatment including surgery, chemotherapy, and radiation treatments can render them temporarily or permanently infertile *and* can result in a sudden menopause. You take a double blow.

Chemotherapy with high doses of long duration, such as that for Hodgkin's disease, will usually result in permanent cessation of ovarian function. Lower chemotherapy doses and shorter treatment courses are generally used for breast cancer, so there may only be temporarily interruption of ovarian function. Ovarian cycles may return after a few months, but in spite of this successful pregnancies are less frequent than normal because of ovarian damage from chemotherapy.

The same is true for radiation therapy, unless the irradiation is directed into the pelvis. In that case, the ovaries are usually destroyed. For pelvic and abdominal irradiation, the ovaries can sometimes be protected by shielding them with lead aprons. Other attempts have been to surgically relocate them out of the pelvis near the colon at the time of hysterectomy. This is called *ovarian transposition*. Dr. D. D. Feeny studied 200 women treated for cervical cancer with preservation of the ovaries and surgical transposition. He found that 50% of those who had radiation therapy experienced ovarian failure within 24 months, in spite of the transposition (Feeny 1995). So, the answers are not at hand for how to conserve fertility and normal hormone production with radiation treatment of pelvic cancers.

Some work has been done on collecting ova before surgery or chemotherapy and storing them for later use after cancer therapy is completed. The idea has been to fertilize the ova with the partner's sperm and implant them into the uterus or fallopian tubes. There are many technical problems including hormonal support of the pregnancy, but it has worked for some women. This is the same procedure that you may have seen reported on TV whereby menopausal women have achieved successful pregnancies.

The emotional trauma of having cancer and the additional blow of lost fertility and/or premature menopause make for a psychic double whammy for women. Pre- and posttreatment counseling are of major importance to women who sustain these enormous bodily changes.

Estrogen replacement therapy is available to most women who choose it, unless their type of cancer has many estrogen receptor sites. In this situation, estrogen use could result in growth of any tumor cells that may remain after treatment and is therefore inadvisable. Breast cancer is an example of such an exception. Hormone replacement is usually appropriate for cervical, vulvar, vaginal, and ovarian cancer. Opinion on HRT after endometrial cancer is divided.

Premature Menopause

Spontaneous premature menopause is a poorly understood phenomenon. It is generally defined as ovarian failure before age 40. It can happen as early as the teens but usually is seen one to two decades later than that. The incidence is about 1% of the female population in the United States.

Heredity seems to be a factor, since women who experience premature menopause commonly have mothers or grandmothers who have done so as well. A damaged X chromosome inherited from either the father or mother is the cause. Family history of premature menopause is not a reliable predictor for any given woman, but, with that kind of a background, delaying a family is probably not a good idea.

Ovaries can be damaged during fetal life by maternal problems such as viral diseases. The growing ovaries may never achieve the usual number of egg cells, so they dwindle prematurely when the female fetus is a grown woman.

Certain autoimmune disorders such as Addison's disease or disseminated lupus erythematosis may result in antibody production, which has an adverse effect on the ovaries or thyroid. They cause premature menopause.

A hysterectomy with conservation of ovaries may also result in premature menopause, but it is quite uncommon for this to happen prior to age 40. Chemotherapy and radiation therapy can do it. Women who live at high altitudes also have earlier menopause.

Smoking is known to be associated with an earlier than usual menopause. This is most likely to occur two to three years before age 51. Rarely, it can happen as much as 10 years short of the average menopausal age. The cause is not certain, but Dr. Wulf Utian, a recognized expert in menopause, says the theories are

1. toxins in tobacco smoke result in the liver altering estrogen such that it is not useful
2. nicotine, a known blood vessel constrictor, reduces blood flow to the ovaries sufficiently over time so that they become atrophic (Utian 1990)

This is just one more reason to be a nonsmoker, and a sure-fire reason if your family history is one of shortened childbearing years.

Diagnosis of spontaneous premature menopause is commonly delayed because the symptoms are more gradual and of milder intensity than those of natural menopause at age 51. The delay is also facilitated by the low index of suspicion on the part of both the young woman who is prematurely menopausal and her physician. The search for the cause of her symptoms may be easily misdirected. The diagnostic test is to check the FSH levels.

Treatment for premature menopause involves hormone replacement therapy. It is much more urgent to strongly recommend HRT in premature menopause. These women have many more postmenopausal years ahead of them than women whose menopause is at the natural age. Heart disease and osteoporosis may foreshorten life significantly, so alternative therapies, which have not been shown to prevent these problems, are not a good recommendation (Ravnikar 1990). As for duration of HRT, lifelong use is as appropriate for premature menopause as for natural menopause. The minimum duration should be through age 51. Then, consider where you wish to go after that, just as in natural menopause. But, keep in mind that the answer to, How long should I stay on HRT? is, As long as you desire the benefits.

Summing Up

It doesn't require any imagination to understand the emotional turmoil experienced by women in whom childbearing capability has been prematurely ended. It may be particularly excruciating if she has not yet become a mother.

The newer technologies mentioned above for in vitro fertilization and hormonal support of a pregnancy offer hope. Nevertheless, these young women are still subject to a menagerie of negative emotions ranging from embarrassment and outrage, to loss of self-esteem and concern that they will become the American stereotypic image of postmenopausal women—an asexual, wrinkled, and wizened old woman. It is therefore of paramount importance that these women seek help and support and that those whose help and support is sought treat them with all the tenderness and compassion that their situation deserves. Becoming properly and fully informed may rely on education by the personal physician, from a menopause clinic, or from a university program. Spouses and peers obviously have major roles to play, as well.

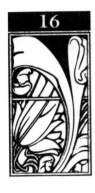

GETTING THE
RIGHT CARE
USER-FRIENDLY HEALTH CARE

Here you will be advised on how to find the health care adviser best for you at midlife. You will learn how to find out if the doctor is qualified to advise you on menopause and related issues and how to interview such a person. The components of an adequate health checkup are discussed.

Health Care Delivery in America

As our health care system continues to change, the solo doctor is gradually going the way of the dinosaur. Medical practice is getting increasingly consolidated into HMOs (health maintenance organizations), PPOs (preferred provider organizations), IPOs (independent practice organizations), and other groupings. *Provider* is the ascendant and politically correct term to describe the person who used to be called the doctor or a physician. *Family doctor* has been replaced with *primary care provider,* and *general practitioner* is an extinct term. The term *practitioner* or *provider* now encompasses physicians, osteopaths, nurses, psychologists, physician's assistants, physical therapists, naturopaths, homeopaths, herbalists, acupuncturists, chiropractors, dietitians, counselors of all types, and others.

The results of all this grouping and consolidating of terms have been less personalized delivery of health care and less regard by the public for health care givers of all stripes. Specialization has been a major contributor. Health care providers in group settings are becoming more and more nine to five types, with the on-call provider providing the providee (you) any 5 P.M. to 9 A.M. services you may require. Emergency rooms and/or urgent care centers are becoming the primary interface for people and the health care system.

As a menopausal woman who wants to know something about your situation, or who wants management for it, you are faced with an astonishing array of practitioners to whom you might turn. Should you see a cardiologist about postmenopausal heart disease? an orthopedist about osteoporosis? an endocrinologist about hormones? a gynecologist about uterine bleeding or vaginal dryness? a sex therapist about painful sex? a chiropractor for a backache? a psychologist about mood shifts? a gerontologist about aging? What a menu.

The consensus among governmental bureaucracies, insurance companies, and health care groups is that everyone should be assigned, or choose, a primary care provider (PCP). Your PCP is then responsible for assessing your problem and providing your care or referring you to someone who can. In most settings, you still have a choice as to who will be your primary care provider. For women, it can be a family practitioner, an internist, or an obstetrician/gynecologist. That certainly narrows it down somewhat.

DO YOUR HOMEWORK FIRST

For you to get optimal health care as a midlife woman, you have a responsibility to yourself to know what that is. The health care system evolving in our country is continuing to de-emphasize "going the extra mile" for patients and is increasingly in the hands of the bottom line medical economists, the bean counters. Physicians are no longer the sole decision makers as to what care you get or when you get it. This means you must be more proactive, involved, and knowledgeable about your own health needs. Your chances of getting the advice and care you need when you see your doctor will be enhanced if you have an advance appreciation of what is right for you. You can prepare an agenda of your questions and concerns from what you have learned about midlife health; this should be communicated to your doctor. If you are obviously informed on these issues, you will much more likely be listened to—and heard.

To do this, consider making up a checklist of your personal risk factors for health problems you may face at midlife and beyond. Such a risk inventory is a means not only of informing yourself, but also for alerting your doctor to potential future problems. Table 16-1 is a guideline for you to use. Circle the risk factors that pertain to you. Some of the lifestyle risk factors can be altered favorably, such as smoking, alcohol consumption, obesity, and a sedentary life. Others that are family traits are just the genetic cards you have been dealt, and you're just stuck with those. Still, knowing what risks you face can alert you and your doctor to appropriate advice about lifestyle changes and a screening plan to pick up potential problems at an early stage.

Table 16-1

RISK FACTORS CHECK SHEET

Disease or condition	Lifestyle influence of risk	Family inheritance of risk	Risk from current or prior disorder
Heart disease	Estrogen deficiency, smoking, obesity, high fat diet, sedentary lifestyle	Coronary disease before 65 in female 1st-degree relatives; before 55 in 1st-degree male relatives	High blood lipids, diabetes, high blood pressure
Obesity	High fat diet, sedentary lifestyle	Lifelong obesity in 1st- or 2nd-degree relatives	Hypothyroidism, diabetes, insulin resistance
Osteoporosis	Estrogen deficiency, prolonged absence of menses, low calcium intake, smoking, sedentary lifestyle, excess alcohol, prolonged thyroid drug or steroid use	1st-degree relative with osteoporosis, Caucasian with light skin, Asian	Hypoparathyroidism
Diabetes	Obesity	1st- or 2nd-degree relative with diabetes, Native American, African American, Hispanic	High blood lipids, high blood pressure, gestational diabetes
Breast cancer	High fat diet, obesity, delayed pregnancies or none, smoking, excess alcohol, sedentary lifestyle	1st- and 2nd-degree relatives under age 50 with breast cancer, strong family history of colorectal, breast, ovarian cancer	Prior cancer of breast, ovary, colon
Lung cancer	Smoking, asbestos exposure		Chronic lung diseases: emphysema, bronchitis
Colorectal cancer	High fat, low fiber diet, sedentary lifestyle	1st- or 2nd-degree relatives with colorectal cancer under age 55, familial polyposis, strong family history of other cancers	Prior polyps or colon cancer, prior breast or ovarian cancer
Uterine cancer	Unopposed estrogen use, prolonged anovulation, obesity, hypertension		Polycystic ovary syndrome (PCO)
Ovarian cancer	No term pregnancies, high fat diet, smoking, talcum-asbestos use, long-term fertility drugs(?)	1st- and 2nd-degree relatives with ovarian cancer, 1st- or 2nd-degree relatives with ovarian or breast cancer, strong family history of other cancers	Prior breast or colon cancer
Cervical cancer	Sexually transmitted disease, early sexual activity, smoking		Prior high grade cellular abnormality (HGSIL) or cancer, HPV or herpes infection
Thyroid cancer	X-ray irradiation of thyroid, face, neck	1st- and 2nd-degree relatives with thyroid or autoimmune disease	Prior autoimmune disease

Table 16-2
SCREENING TESTS AND EXAMINATIONS FOR WOMEN OVER AGE 40

Exam or test	Over 40	Specific age	If at high risk
Complete physical exam teeth to toes	Annual		Annual or patient/physician judgment
Blood tests:			
Complete blood count	Every 5 years	Annual over 65	Annual with history of anemia
Lipid panel	Every 3–5 years if normal	Every 1–3 years over 65	Twice yearly
Fasting blood sugar	Every 3–5 years		Annual if at risk for diabetes
Gynecological tests:			
Pap screening	Every 2 years if 3 consecutive yearly smears normal	Start late teens or earlier if having sex	Annual if high grade cellular lesion or at risk for cancer
Sexually transmitted disease: GC, HIV, chlamydia, syphilis, herpes, HPV			Any time if exposed HIV test both partners before and 6 months after new sexual relationship
Pelvic ultrasound			Any time for unknown pelvic mass or postmenopausal bleeding to measure endometrium
			Patient discretion if at risk for ovarian cancer and/or on HRT
Breast screening:			
Self exam		Monthly starting in late teens	
Physician exam	Annual	1–3 years, age 16–39	
Mammogram (MGM)	Annual after 40		Earlier if high risk
Genetic screening			1st- and 2nd-degree relatives under 50 with breast cancer 2 or more relatives with ovarian cancer at any age 1 relative with breast cancer *plus* 1 with ovarian cancer
Ultrasound			Any time for unknown mass or back-up for mammogram mass
High definition ultrasound imaging			Backup for suspicious MGM lesion before biopsy
Magnetic resonance imaging (MRI)			Backup for suspicious lesion before biopsy or lumpectomy

Table 16-2 (continued)

Exam or test	Over 40	Specific age	If at high risk
Cardiovascular:			
Blood pressure check	2 or more/year		Patient/physician judgment
Electrocardiogram	Baseline at 40	Every 5 years over 40	Annual if at high risk
Treadmill ECG		Baseline at 50	Every 3 years Anytime if have angina
Colorectal screening:			
Fecal occult blood test, 3-day stool sample			Yearly if flexible sigmoidoscopy or colonoscopy not locally available
Flexible sigmoidoscopy		Every 5 years after 50	
Colonoscopy		10 years younger than youngest 1st- or 2nd-degree relative with colon cancer under age 55	Every 5 years with risk factors After positive 3-day occult blood test
Osteoporosis screening:			
DEXA bone density scan			Baseline at 40 if at risk Every 2–3 years if not on HRT after menopause Every 2 years if on medication for severe osteoporosis
Thyroid screening:			
TSH	Every 2 years		Annual if high risk or have symptoms
Other tests:			
Chest X-ray			Annual for smokers or patient/physician judgment
Urinalysis		Annual after 50	
Ca-125			Annual after menopause if high risk for ovarian cancer
Immunizations:			
Tetanus-diphtheria		Booster every 10 years	
Influenza vaccine		Yearly after 55	Patient/physician judgment for chronic lung disease Yearly for health workers
Hepatitis B			Health workers, travel in China or SE Asia, other specific exposure risks, children
Hepatitis A		Travelers	
Measles, mumps, and rubella (German measles)			Repeat if initial shot after 1973 since weak vaccines used

After you have assessed your risk factors, look over Table 16-2 for a schedule of examinations and tests that may apply to your particular situation as a midlife woman with your personal risk factors. This table represents a consensus of many current opinions of how to keep track of your health. Regard it as a guideline, as opposed to a cookbook of health management. This should be part of your discussion with your midlife health care adviser. A plan for current and future health monitoring can evolve from the information you present to your doctor from Tables 16-1 and 16-2.

Once you are armed with some valuable background information about yourself, you are ready to seek out the health care adviser who can integrate your data into a coordinated plan for getting you into your next third of life in the best possible health.

Finding the Right Doc—or Provider, or Practitioner

Now you must find one who is user-friendly regarding midlife care in general and perimenopausal-menopausal care specifically. The best way to proceed is to first inform yourself as much as possible about menopause. This can be done by reading books like this one and others, plus attending lectures and seminars, watching videos and TV specials, and investigating support groups and other sources. With this background, choosing the provider most suitable for you will be easier. Your goal should be to select someone knowledgeable about menopause. You should be looking for a doctor with whom you can form a partnership. It should be one who values your input and questions about your health, and someone who perceives their role as a teacher and health counselor. It also should be someone with whom you can feel confident as well as comfortable, and with whom you feel a good chance exists of establishing mutual respect.

Locating this paragon usually turns out to be a word-of-mouth process. Probably the best source is the recommendation of another doctor whom you trust. It also can be helpful to contact the head of the Ob/Gyn Department of a local hospital or the president of the hospital medical staff. Once you have a recommendation, find out if that doctor has privileges to practice at a hospital that is reputable and convenient.

Should you choose a gynecologist? My experience is that you should have a gynecologist as well as a family physician or internist. Gynecologists are much more likely to have kept up with menopausal developments in this rapidly changing field. They will also be more attuned to other situations common to midlife such as breast lumps, osteoporosis, gynecologic screening, vaginal infections, sexual problems, and menstrual irregularity.

Lists, directories, and yellow pages can give you names, addresses, and phone numbers, but one of the best references is personal experience—yours or someone else's. Decide first if your health care adviser is to be a gynecologist, an internist, a holistic practitioner, or an alternative health care provider and find out as much as you can about that person. The county medical society can help. Various boards, registries and licensing bureaus may have information, but most of this will be rather generic. If you cannot locate someone who has direct experience with the doctor you choose, you'll need to do it on your own.

THE INTERVIEW

One of the first clues may come when you make an appointment. Do they give good phone? Were you treated courteously? Can you get an appointment? Is it before next year? Establish clearly that you wish to interview the doctor (or provider as you prefer) about menopause: this is an *interview*, not a workup. Same thing if this is your established doctor. Make a list of the questions to which you need answers, and prioritize them. Don't make the list so long that the two of you will need to send out for food before you can cover everything. Organize your thoughts in advance and state them clearly at the start of the interview. If you are interrupted during your statement (a common failing among doctor or provider types), then be assertive and say you haven't finished yet. Your responsibility in this relationship is to be sure your doctor has listened to you and heard you. Don't be rude, but neither be timid. Insist on lay language and ask for an explanation for any medical lingo you do not understand. Press for direct answers to your questions; don't settle for talking "around" your question. If it has not been answered, ask it again. You will feel more confident and at ease if you are fully clothed during this interview. Do not be bullied by office personnel who insist you cannot do it this way because it is not "routine." Point out that you have come for an interview, not an exam.

As your interchange is under way, start assessing the doctor as to whether he/she is friendly and approachable, as opposed to disinterested, arrogant, or hostile. Does this doctor seem to care about you? Caring and empathy are hallmarks of sensitive people. This bodes well for a good doctor/patient relationship, especially where menopause is concerned. Be alert to evaluating this doctor's attitude toward perimenopause and menopause by listening to what is said about hot flashes, moodiness, memory lapses, etc., and *how* it is said.

+ Indifference: "Don't worry about hot flashes. They're a natural part of menopause and they'll go away."
+ Condescension: "There, there now (maybe with a pat on the head, or shoulder), you're too young to be menopausal."

♦ Hostile: "Well tie a string to the blasted car keys, and hang 'em around your neck."

Find out if the doctor advocates HRT and, if so, what regimens would be suggested for you to use. What is the response to your opposition to HRT, or to your interest in alternative therapies? Was postmenopausal heart disease or osteoporosis mentioned? How about this doctor's concern and knowledge about fitness and diet?

If you are satisfied that your interviewee is up to speed on menopause and you feel this doctor will relate to you, your menopausal concerns, and your overall life, then you've got a winner. If not, try another. You may also be able to locate a menopause specialist near you by getting a recommendation from the

North American Menopause Society
4074 Abingdon Road
Cleveland, OH 44106
(216) 844-3334, fax (216) 844-3348

What Should I Be Checked For?

A midlife health assessment can be incorporated into your annual examination. It should cover the health components that relate to perimenopause and menopause. Certain conditions are more prevalent in perimenopausal women. These should be identified early in order to initiate intervention and, thus, avoid a deleterious effect on you when you become menopausal.

You should have a complete medical history taken, especially if you have a new doctor. Also get a complete physical examination, selected laboratory tests as suggested in Table 16-2, and any appropriate immunizations.

♦ A *complete medical history* should include any family history of CVD, osteoporosis, cancer, diabetes, thyroid disease, mental illness, Alzheimer's disease, and obesity. Your personal history should cover your current health status, including any menopausal symptoms. Dietary and nutritional status, plus exercise activities, should be evaluated. You should disclose use, or abuse, of alcohol, tobacco, or drugs. Sexual practices such as single or multiple partners are relevant, as are psychosocial factors like marital status, family dynamics, occupation, stress, anxiety, and depression.
♦ Your *physical examination* should record your height, weight, and blood pressure. The exam should specifically include your mouth and teeth, neck (thyroid and lymph glands), heart and lungs, breasts and

axillae (armpits for lymph glands), abdomen, skin, and pelvic area (with rectovaginal exam).

+ *Laboratory studies* should include a lipid panel (every 5 years for cholesterol, HDL, LDL, triglycerides), mammogram (annually after 40), sigmoidoscopy (every 5 years after 50).

+ *Immunization* recommendations may be tetanus (every 10 years) and influenza vaccine (yearly starting at 55). Hepatitis and pneumonia immunizations should be based on individual risk factors.

Certain screening tests may be recommended for some conditions depending on risk factors you may have.

+ *Thyroid disease*, especially an underactive thyroid, is common in women. It is important to avoid overtreatment if you are menopausal because this enhances osteoporosis. Annual to biannual monitoring with a thyroid stimulating hormone (TSH) test should be done.

+ *Diabetes* is well known to enhance the risk of CVD, and together with menopause it's a double whammy. Annual screening should be done if you have a family history of diabetes, body weight greater than 20% above ideal weight, or a history of diabetes during pregnancy.

+ *High blood pressure* after age 50 is more common in women than in men. It is more common in African-American women than women of other races. Risk factors to look for are a previous history of hypertension, a family history of CVD especially if at an early age, heavy sodium (salt) or alcohol use, smoking, coronary artery disease, chronic kidney disease, prior stroke, high cholesterol, diabetes, obesity, and chronic stress. Monitoring your blood pressure at more frequent intervals is advisable, as well as measures to control the risk factors that are correctable.

+ *Pap tests* are recommended every three years after three consecutive annual tests are normal. Recent studies in Denmark, Norway, Canada, and the United States all show that lower levels of cervical cancer are seen when the screening interval is every two years. There is no significant difference between one- and two-year intervals, but the cancer rate is up to four times higher if it is every three years. It is apparent from these studies that the existing recommendation for Pap screening every three years should be changed to two years. Some large medical groups are stopping Pap screening of women in their late 60s to early 70s. This is advisable only if you have never had an abnormal Pap smear *and* if you have not had any of the following risk factors for cervical cancer: multiple sex partners, started sex at an early age, had herpes in the past, are a cigarette smoker, have had a human papilloma virus (HPV) infection. HPV is seen in almost all cervical cancers. Since 25% of cervical cancer and 40% of deaths from it are seen in women over age 65, many of these will be missed if screening is stopped.

✦ *Occult blood testing of feces* starting at age 50 to screen for colorectal cancer has been an annual recommendation for many years. Many doctors used to check a stool sample from an examining glove after a rectal exam. The glove sample produces far too many false positive results, and this exam has been abandoned. To be accurate, the three-day test (stool sample on three consecutive days) must be preceded by a full week of dietary restriction plus the three days of stool sample collection. This means no red meats, raw fruits (especially melons), raw veggies (especially radishes, turnips, horseradish), aspirin, nonsteroidal anti-inflammatory agents (like ibuprofen), and vitamin C. Most people cannot or do not follow the restrictions well enough for reliable results. This test is being abandoned also. The newer recommendation to replace occult blood screening is this: If you have first- or second-degree relatives who have had colon cancer under age 55, you should have a colonoscopy at an age 10 years younger than your relative's age when it was discovered. If everything is normal, your colonoscopy should be repeated every five years. If there is no colorectal disease in your family, a colonoscopy or flexible sigmoidoscopy should be done every 5 years starting at age 50. At this point in time, these exams are not available in all communities. In this situation, the three-day test for occult blood should be done annually starting at age 50.

Summing Up

With the changes that are taking place in the health care delivery system in our country, it is increasingly important and necessary for all of us to be more informed about our health and to be more proactive in its management. We are all still dependent on health care professionals for the application of expertise, but we must assume at least part of the responsibility for getting the appropriate care. This chapter has been about just one of those responsibilities, namely the locating of a health adviser who is qualified to provide you with information, advice, and management of perimenopausal and menopausal concerns. The coming years are too important for you to have anything less than a competent and compassionate doctor.

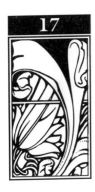

JUST FOR MEN: ANDROPAUSE AND MENOPAUSE

READ THIS GUYS.
IT TAKES TWELVE MINUTES

These next pages will cover midlife changes for men, plus a summary of perimenopause and menopause for men to read. Included will be strategies for making the transition easier for both of you.

Andropause

Male menopause is a term that is quite frequently used to describe midlife changes in men, although when you stop to think that menopause means the cessation of menstrual periods, the term *male menopause* becomes patently ridiculous—a genuine oxymoron. Changes in men *do* occur with advancing age that have a negative impact on such functions as physical and athletic prowess, memory, sex, sleep, and productivity. They are very gradual—they occur over 30 to 40 years—and in no way do they compare with the abrupt changes in women. This is not to say that midlife crises do not happen to men. They do indeed occur, just as in women, but they differ. In their book *Managing Your Menopause*, Dr. Wulf Utian and Ruth Jacobowitz succinctly express the difference as a "crisis of performance" for men versus a "crisis of appearance" for women. For example:

✦ At midlife a man will need glasses to read a menu, he can't beat his son at tennis anymore, marathon sex is but a memory, and the giant sucking sound each morning is when he is buttoning his trousers.

- For women, there is a daily "smile line" check, firm breasts and a tight fanny are goners, half of her wardrobe only half fits, and whether or not to color those wisps of gray is an ongoing internal debate, as well as the issue of "sensible clothes."

IT'S HORMONAL, BY GOLLY

It is well established that men have a decline in hormone production of both *testosterone* and *growth hormone*. Most American men do not know this. This decline is a climacteric, just as in women. Hers is over five to 10 years, while his spans three decades or more. Testosterone starts diminishing at about age 40, but significant drops are not recorded until after about 60. In Europe, the male climacteric is a better understood and more widely accepted concept. It is referred to as *andropause*, a word patterned after *menopause* and incorporating *androgen*. Androgens are male hormones, such as testosterone. Study of male hormone deficiency is getting under way in the United States, but recommendations for replacement therapy lie well into the future.

The physical effects of male hormone withdrawal are usually manifested by age 60. Men become aware of decreased muscle mass and strength, altered sexual capability, and diminished vitality. Osteoporosis is even a possibility.

The emotional effects of andropause include moodiness, diminished concentration, lessened assertiveness, damaged self-image, diminished self-esteem, an altered outlook on life, and perhaps a negative assessment of goal accomplishments. A man's self-identity is tied up with physical ability, sexual prowess, occupational success, and societal impact. Since all of these may be changing for him at midlife, andropause constitutes a grave threat to his perception of his manhood.

Outside factors influence a man's emotional status at midlife. His wife may be perimenopausal or postmenopausal, which suggests to him that time is marching on for him as well. He may have risen as far as he will ever get in his occupation. In today's marketplace, continued employment may well be an uncertainty. Teenage children can be just as stressful for men as for women, and the same goes for when they have flown the nest, or want to return to the roost. Aging parent responsibilities may intrude.

As the contemplation of midlife is undertaken, a man may have serious regrets—that he was not successful enough in his occupation, did not make enough money to provide well for his family, neglected his wife and the kids too much, didn't have enough sex with his wife (or other women), did have sex with other women and damaged his marriage. The list may be endless. All of this introspection can lead a man onto either of two paths. He may try to start it all over again with a new partner. The "trophy wife" is a common enough story in our culture. Or, his years may have conferred upon him enough wisdom to make him more appreciative of life as it happens, resulting in his becoming a more sensitive and nurturing person.

So, at midlife change happens. Call it andropause, call it male menopause, call it a midlife crisis as you please, but transformation is the process we are talking about. It is a transition, a stage, a phase, a passage that has its roots in hormone depletion and aging. As with women, it can be successfully navigated with knowledge about what is happening, with communication about feelings, and at some future time it may be aided by hormone replacement therapy (see Chapter 10).

Menopause and Men's Role

Female menopause and men's involvement in it is an important part of this book. Much of what follows will be a reiteration of topics already covered, but slanted toward the goal of male understanding. It won't make all of you men experts on menopause, but you will know enough of the basics to put you way ahead of the curve relative to other men. While you will probably be regarded as on the cutting edge by women acquaintances, you will be regarded as a KISHA (knight in shining armor) by your partner.

CHANGES IN HER BODY AND HER EMOTIONS

Menopause happens to all women. It is utterly unavoidable. At birth, a female infant has all the eggs in her ovaries she is ever going to have; these get gradually depleted with time. By her 40s, very few remain, and this causes a reduction in the effective female hormone production of estrogen and progesterone. The result is a cascade of symptoms and bodily changes including moodiness, hot flashes, vaginal dryness, loss of sleep, decreased sexual desire, poor control of a full bladder, irregular menstrual periods and, eventually, cessation of menstrual periods at about age 51. This takes place over about three to five years, but it may take six to 10 years for a few. All of these symptoms and body changes do not happen to every woman, but it is important for you to know that she has no control over which ones may happen to her. She may be as surprised as you to see and feel the symptoms that show up.

Menopause represents the end of the childbearing era for your partner, a major life event for a woman. It marks the beginning of the next third of life. It is a transition period of fluctuating emotions that typically starts in the mid-40s, and occasionally earlier for some. During the transition, she may seem less self-assured to you because she is in unfamiliar territory, but she will indeed emerge from this passage with new confidence, ready for your future together.

WHAT'S BOTHERING HER

In addition to the physical changes from hormone depletion, her emotional status may be influenced by other factors impinging on her life at this time such as the following:

+ problems *you* might be having with your health, your work, unemployment, or retirement
+ doubts about her continued sexual attractiveness to you
+ anxiety about what it will be like with the children gone from your home, or wanting to return
+ worries about your parents' health
+ concern about her own aging
+ fear of postmenopausal heart disease, the number one cause of death for women after menopause. Within six months after menopause, lack of estrogen causes a rise in LDL (bad cholesterol) and a decrease of HDL (good cholesterol). This puts her at greater risk of a heart attack in later years; prevention needs to start now
+ concern about osteoporosis, or bone loss, which accelerates rapidly after menopause. This is the process that makes little old ladies who are bent and frail. Their bones break easily, which may result in chronic pain, or even premature death. Prevention of osteoporosis needs to start now as well
+ questions about which options she should select to manage her menopause and prevent hormone loss from damaging her body

SEXUAL CHANGE

Menopause can affect your sex life. About 9% of women have an increased sexual desire after menopause. It may derive from factors like freedom from pregnancy worries and no kids in the house. Others find that vaginal dryness and vaginal atrophy (thinning and loss of elasticity) caused by hormone depletion result in painful sex. That can put a real damper on her eagerness to romp about in bed with you, and if you know that sex is hurting her, you also may be reluctant to frolic and gambol in ways sexual.

KEEPING SEX ON LINE

A variety of modalities can alter this favorably for the two of you. Estrogen therapy in the form of tablets, skin patches, vaginal cream, or an estrogen-containing vaginal ring is quite reliable in restoring vaginal moisture and elasticity. Lubricants are very helpful. Even regular sexual stimulation about twice per week helps dryness. One of the very best protectors of sexuality is to talk with each other about your sexual needs and sexual problems. It isn't easy for many people, but the payoff in better sex can be enormous. If you are experiencing diminished erection firmness and duration, let her know that more penile stimulation before sex can be helpful. She may tell you that natural lubrication of her vagina is quite possible but that it requires a longer period of foreplay than all those years ago when you were both sex bombs. Menopause and andropause do not constitute a valid reason to assume the end of sex is at hand. The game is still the same, but the techniques for playing it have changed a little.

SHE MAY SEEM WEIRD

Your wife's emotional profile will likely change during her transition through menopause. She may look perfectly healthy to you but she may feel absolutely rotten. The confident, competent, and in-control woman you have been accustomed to may become anxious and insecure. Now she is shooting rats with cannons, as minor irritants provoke uncharacteristically harsh responses. She may be utterly destroyed by criticism. One day she seems normal, and the next she's so down and depressed, she can hardly get out of her own way. It may seem at times that she is mentally ill, but there is actually, at this stage of life, less of the serious illness called major depression than there is in younger women. So don't worry that she may need to taken off to "the home."

Your salvation, and hers too, will be assured if you keep these thoughts at the forefront of your mind.

+ She cannot prevent this emotional roller coaster because her hormonal disequilibrium is not in her control.
+ It is temporary. Her volatility is not permanent. Tranquillity and new self-assurance await her completion of the transition.
+ Coping with this phase requires effort and understanding on your part, but you will ultimately find it worthwhile for you both.

SHE HAS SOME CHOICES

There are things she can do to help, some of which require some thoughtful study and sober decision making. Hormone replacement therapy (HRT), while not for everyone for medical and/or philosophical reasons, can be remarkably effective in controlling the body changes and emotional upheavals. HRT also helps reduce the risk of heart disease and prevents osteoporosis for the large majority of women. Alternative therapies also exist including herbal medicines, homeopathy, acupuncture, and a variety of stress management strategies. Some of these latter treatment options are not well grounded in reliable science as yet, but many women are helped considerably by them. All of these management choices have risks associated with them, varying from health risks to the risk of ineffectiveness. *But,* doing nothing at all carries a much more serious risk, since menopause poses its own serious health threats. Other sources of important help to her are a low fat diet, a good fitness program, stopping smoking, and minimizing alcohol consumption.

YOU'VE GOT SOME IMPORTANT CHOICES TOO

There are things you can do to help. Most important, perhaps, is that she needs you to be there for her. She needs to know you understand that she has little control of the changes happening to her body. You cannot solve the myriad problems confronting your partner, but if you are supportive and even tempered, her chances of successfully coping with them are greatly improved. Remember that she is having a crisis of appearance. Reassure her that you find her attractive. Warm, honest hugs (lots of them) say volumes about how you feel toward her. Listen to her attentively as she mulls over what treatment options might be best for her. Your opinion might even be solicited if she feels you have done some homework.

FITNESS IS EXTREMELY IMPORTANT FOR YOUR PARTNER AT MIDLIFE

Exercise is a great elevator of mood and helps considerably with hot flashes. Aerobic exercise for 30 minutes, 3–5 times weekly will produce cardiovascular fitness in anyone. It also helps prevent osteoporosis. You will do her a great service by encouraging her to start a fitness program. And by the way, pal, you could probably use some huffing and puffing yourself, so why don't you offer to exercise *with* her? You don't need to put on a thong leotard and go to aerobic dance class, although you would be quite welcome, but the two of you can do aerobic walking together (45–60 minutes, 3–5 times per week). Jogging works too, but it's very hard on your body. My wife and I regularly solve the world's problems, as well as our own, four to five times a week during brisk walking. A healthy diet is another component of fitness that is a necessity for her and will benefit you both. A low fat diet protects you from heart disease, the number one killer for both of you. The more you emphasize vegetables, fruits, pastas, and grains, the healthier you will be. If you get into cooking and marketing with her, you may find a new stimulus that brings you closer to each other. Just think of diet and exercise as life insurance.

HER MOOD SWINGS

You can help with her mood swings. You can't prevent them, but you can avoid aggravating them by asking her to let you know when she is feeling out of sorts. In her book *The Pause*, Dr. Lonnie Barbach calls this tactic "getting a weather report." If it's a stormy day for her and you want to inquire about a previously unexplained new dent in the car, write it down and defer the discussion for calmer times—one or two days max. After a day or two, it may not be a big deal for you anymore, and you can delete it from the agenda, especially if you now remember that *you* did it when you ran over your kid's bicycle. This doesn't mean that you have to swallow your words for fear of her wrath every time you have concerns. You have rights and needs also. It just makes it more probable that you will have a productive discussion if she is not having a bad day.

If she *is* having a day where she is shooting rats with cannons because you left your shoes in the living room again, Barbach suggests that you divide the intensity of her reaction by a factor of 10. Then, admit to the underlying validity of her complaint (you *did* leave those damn shoes there) and withdraw from the battlefield. Nothing productive is accomplished by your angrily pointing out her exaggerated objection to your minor indiscretion. Later, when she has regained her composure, she will appreciate your understanding.

Summing Up

From all of the above, I hope you realize that, as a man, you have immense power to make an enormous difference for a woman in the menopausal transition. Some friction and conflict is inevitable, of course, but you will likely find that successfully dealing with it will inaugurate new growth for you as a couple.

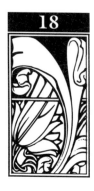

THE NEXT THIRD
FREE AT LAST

Here is the point toward which I have been directing you during this entire book. As you read this final chapter, my hope is that you will see that menopause is the beginning of your new life, your new era—what Gail Sheehy calls your "second adulthood" (Sheehy 1995).

Women in America and other industrialized societies are not rewarded for having arrived at the postreproductive era of life. In many less complex cultures, women rise to high levels of esteem and reverence after menopause. Our perception of the postmenopausal woman is that she is no longer young, so how can she possibly have any worth or credibility? Her image was established by prior generations whose postmenopausal women wore their hair in a bun, donned frumpy clothes, never had a clue about a healthy diet, never even mentioned the word "exercise" let alone did any, felt obligated to abandon sex, and sat invisibly by to await becoming a wrinkled old lady. Today, this negative image still finds willing accomplices in the news media, the film industry, medical literature, and in all of us.

But as this negative caricature took hold, what happened to the real postmenopausal woman? Upon reaching midlife, and especially upon reaching menopause, past American women always started to disappear. It almost seems to have been something of a mutual agreement between the woman who recognized she was no longer young and the rest of the populace who agreed with her. She didn't turn heads anymore. Men stopped flirting and doing all those awkward, silly things they seem to do when confronting an attractive young woman. Her opinion was solicited less and weighted more lightly when given. If she tried to cling to a youthful image with youngish clothes, makeup, and hairstyle, she was derided as garish or pitied as a faded ingenue. It was not credible to think of aging women having sex. Acceptance came only if she sheepishly withdrew from the arena of youthfulness and allowed herself to fade into obscurity. No more red teddys or black negligees. It was now flannel nightgown time. She became socially, sexually, and intellectually invisible.

Carolyn Heilbrun, professor of humanities at Columbia University, sees it differently. She acknowledges that invisibility is indeed inevitable, but it is transitory. Heilbrun has stated that the midlife woman will become invisible until she relearns seeing and forgets about being seen. A young woman is known by how she looks and by who looks at her. A midlife woman is known by what she observes, does, and says.

Embracing this change is a transition, not a concept that just grabs you some morning as you step out of the shower. Sure, it's disappointing to become invisible to people oriented only to youth and invisible to the "male gaze," but that must be dealt with. Dealing with it involves realizing that you must become centered on how *you* feel and on what *you* think. Now is the time to become proactive and to make things happen that *you* want to happen. Now is the time to stop inwardly asking, What will people think? The contemporary midlife woman can, and is, doing this. She is emerging from her transition of invisibility with a new and positive self-perception. The emerging image is that of a confidant woman who does not regret that she is no longer young. A new energy accrues to her that is both physical and intellectual. She is still feminine and still beautiful, but with the inner confidence that derives from wisdom and experience. The packaging may be a little different, but the concept is the same, if not improved.

While the myths and the negative stereotypes still persist in a distressingly large segment of America, CHANGE, it is a comin'. Can you just imagine the contemporary woman, with her established interest in fitness and health, upon becoming menopausal just tying her hair into a grandma bun, trashing her wardrobe, and saying to her partner, "Well Clyde, that rips it for sex." Not a chance. Menopause is coming out of the closet.

Midlife Role Models Exist in Abundance

+ **Marian Anderson** was the first black woman to sing at the New York Metropolitan Opera, and that was a major accolade in 1955. She was 53 years old that January evening.
+ **Margaret Thatcher** became the United Kingdom's prime minister in midlife on the strength of her personal conviction that legislators form consensus and compromises, but leaders lead.

- **Katharine Hepburn, Jessica Tandy,** and **Cicely Tyson** all left their mark on the stage and screen not just before age 50, but *after* as well.
- **Ruth Bader Ginsburg** was turned down as a proposed law clerk by Supreme Court Justice Felix Frankfurter because she was a young woman; now in her 60s, she herself is a Justice on the Supreme Court.
- **Gloria Steinem**'s contribution to the women's revolution is unquestioned. She herself is a one-woman revolution. Her energy continues to flow into her midlife as she addresses self-esteem in her book *Revolution From Within* (Little, Brown 1992). In *Moving Beyond Words* (Simon & Schuster 1994), she says that the past and future are not really important and that there is "no second like this one."
- **Barbara Jordan**'s sonorous voice is now stilled, but hers was a giant presence in American politics, and she was her most influential as a midlife woman.

All of the above women were high profile midlife achievers who are widely known and revered because of their remarkable accomplishments. They probably had hot flashes and troubled sleep and couldn't find their blasted car keys once in a while, but they persevered, resisted invisibility, and flourished. This is happening at the grassroots level too. Think of the midlife women you know who are bank managers, school principals, doctors, mayors, lawyers, business owners, media personalities, grandmothers-of-the-year, waitresses, secretaries, pink ladies at the hospital, and volunteers of all stripes. They too are refusing to become invisible.

The Other Side of the Transition

The disarray of menopausal transition is only temporary. This book has presented a plethora of bad news about menopause, I will admit, but the purpose has been to empower you to successfully manage it and steer a course through it. Transitions are never easy for any of us, but knowledge and preparation always make them smoother. On the other side, a new era begins. You won't be the same as before, because a new perspective will change you forever.

At this point in your life, you can stop being concerned about what other people think and start concentrating on what *you* think. Since your era as a caregiver has come to a close, you can now shift your attention to yourself. No more minivans full of soccer players, no more teeth to straighten, and no more PTA meetings. Set yourself free by recognizing that your identity is no longer based on how you look, or even on how others look *at* you. Youth-oriented cosmetic ads will seem a little silly, because it is no longer necessary for you to look the age they prescribe for you. As a matter of fact, you may feel ennobled by the wrinkles you have earned and the wisdom they paint upon your countenance. Now is the time to set aside any regret for goals you did not accomplish. You are FREE, you have been LIBERATED.

As always in life, there could be some downsides. Your caregiving role may be prolonged by ill parents or an ailing partner. As you are becoming energized by your new self-interest, your older partner may be reigning his energies in. This may strain your relationship until compromises are worked out. You may find yourself without a partner and bewildered as to whether seeking another or living alone is preferable. Seek third-party counseling if these situations seem too much to handle.

Now is the time to allow new goals into your life. There does not need to be any particular limitation placed on your goals based on what post-menopausal women are expected to do "at your age." Neither your mental age nor your biological age need to be related to your chronological age. Climb a mountain if you want to, start a new business, join a health club, do volunteer work, run a marathon, get a new hair color, pursue a hobby, go to college. Don't get really hung up on goal-setting, though. That can scatter you in too many directions. Just keep an open mind and let a new interest wash over you if it will. It will be like a new discovery that you have somehow happened upon, something much more stimulating.

A NEW ROLE

Regard yourself as an active participant in the redefining of women's role at the postmenopausal stage of life. Much can be gleaned from the support of other women, and you, as a seasoned veteran of the menopause struggle, can be an invaluable help to others. Contact women's groups, and help get the word out about menopause. You can attend lectures, give a lecture, write an article, participate in talk radio, start a support group. I hope I don't sound too evangelistic here. I'm not advocating that you get "MENOPAUSAL" tattooed on your forehead, but you must know by now that I think menopause deserves to be better understood, and postmenopausal women, more respected.

START A SUPPORT GROUP

This is easy to do and immensely valuable to participants. Keep it small (maybe 8–12 members) because your interaction will be much freer and more frank than would be the case in a large group. Sheer group size often has an inhibiting effect on free exchange, especially for those women who are basically reticent to discuss being menopausal.

Begin by relating your own experiences and concerns. In time, your group will arrive at a consensus on areas about which you would like to be better informed. Books and other literature can be reviewed, newsletters discussed, and videos played. Check your local library for these things, as well as audiotapes. Invite a guest speaker to address menopause in general or another topic of specific interest like osteoporosis, CVD, sex, fitness, hormone replacement, or alternative management options. Be certain that any guest speakers are experts on their subject. Personal physicians may be well liked, but that doesn't necessarily mean they are up to speed on menopause. On the other hand, your invitation may stimulate your physician to become better informed, which benefits many more than just your group.

Encourage your members to help others such as friends, relatives, coworkers, and partners to become better informed. The more it is talked about, the sooner we will get menopause out of the closet.

The Final Word

Postmenopausal women have been invisible for too long. It is not right for you to be consigned to this outer darkness and expected to find contentment in just being on the right side of the grass. Be of good cheer, for a change is under way, and it is gathering pace as mature women are leaving their mark on our culture at every level. America has not yet conferred full value on postmenopausal women, *but* it is coming.

SUGGESTED READING

American Heart Association. *American Heart Association Low-Salt, Low-Cholesterol Cookbook.* New York: Times Books, 1995. A great book that tells you why and shows you how to have a heart-healthy diet.

Cone, Faye Kitchner. *Making Sense Of Menopause.* New York: Simon & Schuster, 1993. A good, easy-to-read overview of menopause, written in a conversational style.

Connor, Sonja L., M.S., R.D., and William E. Connor, M.D. *The New American Diet System.* New York: Simon & Schuster, 1991. An easy-to-understand book on good nutrition. The authors' cholesterol-saturated fat index (CSI) is a quick reference to selecting the healthiest foods.

Karnicky, Lydia, M.D., Anne Rosenberg, M.D., and Marian Betancourt. *What To Do If You Have Breast Cancer.* New York: Little, Brown & Company, 1995. An up-to-date and well-organized book on the facts about breast cancer and its treatment. This book gets women thinking about the treatment options to be considered and answers the myriad questions that are surfacing.

Love, Susan, M.D., with Karen Lindsey. *Dr. Susan Love's Breast Book.* New York: Addison-Wesley, 1995. This revised edition offers an excellent review of breast disease, with emphasis on prevention.

Ornish, Dean, M.D. *Dr. Dean Ornish's Program for Reversing Heart Disease.* New York: Ballantine Books, 1992. A good book for people with heart disease, as well as an excellent guide on how to protect your heart with good nutrition and exercise.

Reichman, Judith, M.D. *I'm Too Young To Get Old.* New York: Times Books, 1996. An extensive review of midlife health concerns, including menopause. Well researched and written in a conversational style. Contains much more detail than most books on this topic.

Stoppard, Miriam, M.D. *The Magic of Sex: The Book That Really Tells Men about Women and Women about Men.* New York: Dorling Kindersly, Inc., 1991. A comprehensive and sensitive book covering sexuality from the perspective of both genders and emphasizing satisfying sex in long-term relationships.

Ullman, D. *Discovering Homeopathic Medicine for the 21st Century.* Berkeley, Calif.: North Atlantic Books, 1991. A good review of the principles and practices of homeopathy.

RESOURCES FOR MORE INFORMATION

AGING

National Council on Aging
409 Third Street, SW, 2nd Floor
Washington, DC 20024
(800) 424-9046

ALTERNATIVE MEDICINE

Chinese Medicine
AAAOM Referrals
4101 Lake Boone Trail, #201
Raleigh, NC 27607
(919) 787-5181

National Center for Homeopathy
810 North Fairfax, Suite 306
Alexandria, VA 22314
(703) 548-7790

National Institutes of Health
Office of Alternative Medicine
6120 Executive Boulevard
Executive Plaza South, Suite 450
Rockville, MD 20892
(301) 402-2466

CANCER

American Cancer Society
1599 Clifton Road, NE
Atlanta, GA 30329
(800) 227-2345

National Cancer Institute
Bethesda, MD 20205
(800) 422-6237

EXERCISE

American College of Sports
Medicine
P.O. Box 1440
Indianapolis, IN 46202
(317) 637-9200

HEART DISEASE

American Heart Association
7320 Greenville Avenue
Dallas, TX 75231
(800) 242-8721

MEDICINES

Food and Drug Administration
(FDA)
8800 Rockville Pike
Bethesda, MD 20852
(301) 295-8228

MENOPAUSE

North American Menopause Society
4074 Abingdon Road
Cleveland, OH 44106
(216) 844-3334

NATURAL PROGESTERONE

Belmar Pharmacy
Lakewood, CO
(800) 525-9473

Madison Pharmacy
Madison, WI
(800) 558-7046

Women's International Pharmacy
5708 Monona Drive
Madison, WI 53716-3152
(800) 279-5708 or (608) 221-7800

OSTEOPOROSIS

National Osteoporosis Foundation
2100 M Street, NW
Washington, DC 20037
(202) 223-3336

PHYSICIANS' ORGANIZATIONS

American College of Obstetricians and Gynecologists
Office of Public Information
409 Twelfth Street, SW
Washington, DC 20024-2188
(202) 484-3321

American Medical Association
515 North State Street

Chicago, IL 60610
(800) 262-3211

SEXUALITY

American Association of Sex Educators, Counselors, and Therapists
435 Michigan Avenue, Suite 1717
Chicago, IL 60611
(312) 644-0828

Council for Sex Information and Education
2272 Colorado Boulevard, #1228
Los Angeles, CA 90041

WOMEN'S HEALTH

HERS Foundation
(Hysterectomy Educational Resources and Services)
(215) 667-7757

National Institutes of Health Office of Research on Women's Health
Building 1, Room 201
9000 Rockville Pike
Bethesda, MD 20892
(301) 402-1770

National Women's Health Network
1325 G Street, NW
Washington, DC 20005
(202) 347-1140

Women's Health Initiative
Federal Building, Room 6A09
9000 Rockville Pike
Bethesda, MD 20892
(800) 548-6636

GLOSSARY ❧

adrenal glands Two small glands located atop the kidneys, which secrete adrenaline and steroid hormones (cortisol, androstenediol, DHEA).

aerobic exercise Physical activity requiring increased oxygen for prolonged periods, which improves the body's capacity to handle oxygen.

alopecia Abnormal and excessive loss of hair.

amenorrhea Prolonged absence of menstrual periods prior to menopause.

amino acids Chemical molecules the human body uses to make proteins. *Essential amino acids* are eight amino acids that the body cannot synthesize and that must be acquired from food. A *complete protein* contains all essential amino acids (animal/dairy products, grains, legumes, seeds, nuts).

androgenic Natural or synthetic substances that produce masculine changes in the body.

androgens A group of male hormones produced in the adrenal glands and gonads (ovaries and testes) of both sexes.

anemia A blood condition in which there is a deficiency of red blood cells, hemoglobin, or total blood volume.

antioxidant Substances such as vitamins A, C, and E, beta-carotene, and selenium, which protect cells from damage by oxidated free radicals.

atherosclerosis Hardening of the arteries produced by deposits composed of cholesterol, fibrin, and platelets.

atrophy Wasting or thinning of cells, tissues, or organs produced by inadequate blood supply resulting in poor cellular nutrition.

autonomic nervous system A self-controlling and functionally independent segment of the nervous system that regulates activity of the heart, involuntary muscles (intestines, blood vessels), and glands. It has two divisions: *sympathetic* and *parasympathetic*.

benign Noncancerous, or nonmalignant.

bioavailability The degree to which a drug or other substance becomes available to tissues after administration.

bioflavinoids Vitamin C and plant substances that have a beneficial influence on blood vessel walls and lymph channels.

cancer A malignant growth of rapidly multiplying abnormal cells, which may invade surrounding tissues or spread to distant parts of the body.

cardiovascular disease (CVD) Disease of the heart and/or vascular system, including arteries, veins, and capillaries.

cellulite Fatty deposits under the skin, which result in a dimpling or lumpy appearance.

cervix The opening of the uterus that projects into the upper vagina.

chlamydia A sexually-transmitted bacterium that is a common cause of pelvic infection and infertility.

cholesterol A sterol chemical that is the precursor for the body to make sex hormones, adrenal hormones, and bile acids. Cholesterol is a component of all animal fats and oils. In the bloodstream it is carried in three forms: high-density lipoprotein (HDL), *low-density lipoprotein* (LDL), and *very low-density lipoprotein* (VLDL).

climacteric The span of years from the time that female hormones begin to decline through the first few years after menopause.

clitoris The small, elongated erectile body situated at the top of the vulva just below the pubic bone. It is the female equivalent of the male penis. The clitoris has erectile vascular tissue and profuse nerve endings, which make it quite sensitive to tactile stimulation and enhance sexual arousal and orgasm.

combined oral contraceptive pill (OCP) A pill taken daily containing in varying doses estrogen and progestin, which prevent ovulation.

complex carbohydrates Natural carbohydrates combined with fiber, minerals, and other nutrients. Examples of foods containing complex carbohydrates are cereals, grains, beans, pasta, vegetables, fruits, and whole grain breads.

conception Fertilization of the female egg by a sperm.

conjugated estrogen A group of estrogens derived from pregnant mare's urine and used commonly in HRT.

contraindication A medical condition that makes it inadvisable to use a certain medication or medical procedure.

corpus luteum A yellow glandular mass in the ovarian follicle that is formed after the follicle has discharged its ovum (egg). Progesterone is produced by the corpus luteum.

cortisone A steroid hormone produced by the adrenal glands with powerful anti-inflammatory activity.

cryosurgery A method of destroying abnormal tissue with extreme cold using specially designed probes through which a refrigerant is circulated.

CT scan A computerized X-ray scan of consecutive sections of the body.

DEXA (dual energy X-ray absorptiometry) A reliable X-ray scan that uses low dose irradiation to measure bone density.

diuretic Synthetic or natural substances that induce the kidneys to excrete salt and water, relieving fluid retention.

dysfunctional uterine bleeding (DUB) Irregular menstrual bleeding, either too much or too long in duration, usually caused by failure of ovulation.

dysplasia An abnormal deviation in the orderliness of cells. It may be a precursor to cancer.

endocrine glands Glands that secrete hormones directly into the blood-stream or lymphatic channels and exert specific effects on other organs. These include the ovaries, pituitary, hypothalamus, adrenal, thyroid, para-thyroid, pancreas, and pineal glands.

endocrinologist Medical specialist in diseases of endocrine glands and their hormones.

endometrial ablation An operation to destroy the lining tissue of the uterus carried out through a hysteroscope using a laser beam or a heated roller-ball instrument.

endometriosis A painful condition resulting from endometrial (uterine lin-ing) tissue being abnormally located outside the uterus, usually in the pelvis and abdomen. Pain is caused when the endometriotic tissue bleeds during menstrual periods, resulting in local irritation and scarring.

endometrium The lining tissue of the uterus.

epinephrine (adrenaline) A hormone produced primarily in the adrenal glands, but also in certain areas of the brain, that helps the body prepare for and cope with stress. It is the "fight or flight" hormone. Normal levels promote mood elevation, but high levels produce feelings of anxiety or dread.

estradiol (E2) The primary and most potent natural estrogen produced by the ovaries.

estriol (E3) A weak estrogen produced from estradiol and estrone. Detect-able in high concentrations in urine during pregnancy.

estrone (E1) An estrogen weaker than estradiol, but stronger than estriol. It is produced in the ovaries, but mostly derived from estradiol and from androstenediol (a weak androgen) in fat cells. Estrone is metabolically convertible to estradiol and thus represents a reservoir for that hormone.

fallopian tubes Long, slender tubes extending from either side of the uterus to the region of the ovary of the same side. They gather up the egg when it is released from the ovary at midcycle and propel it toward the uterus. Fertilization takes place in the tube, and the fertilized egg is transported to the uterus for implantation. The fallopian tube is also known as the *salpinx*. Surgical removal of a fallopian tube is called *salpingectomy*.

fibroid A benign tumor in the uterus caused by overgrowth of muscle tissue in the uterine wall.

follicle A tiny sac in the ovarian surface which contains a single egg (ovum). Follicle cells produce estrogen, and later after egg release, the follicle is transformed into the corpus luteum where progesterone is produced.

FSH (follicle stimulating hormone) A hormone made by the pituitary gland that stimulates the growth and maturation of ovarian follicles and the production of estrogen.

GnRH (gonadotropin releasing hormone) A hormone produced in the hypothalamus that controls the release of FSH and LH from the pituitary gland. It is secreted about every 90 minutes into blood vessels that connect the hypothalamus to the pituitary gland.

gonadotropin Hormones that target the gonads. FSH and LH are human female examples.

hCG (human chorionic gonadotropin) A hormone produced in pregnancy by the placental cells. Once the fertilized egg has developed and attached to the uterine wall, this hormone can be detected in a pregnancy test.

hormone replacement therapy (HRT) The replacement of female hormones when natural ovarian production has declined or when there has been a loss by any other endocrine gland.

hormones Chemical substances produced by endocrine glands and cells that are carried in the bloodstream to other organs and tissues and exert multiple metabolic effects.

hypertension Elevation of blood pressure.

hypothalamus An endocrine gland situated at the base of the brain. It is regarded as the master control center since it regulates body temperature, appetite, thirst, sleep, sexual desire, and other important body functions. It also regulates the pituitary gland, which in turn governs the other endocrine glands.

hysterectomy Surgical removal of the uterus.

hysteroscope A thin, multichanneled tube with fiberoptic lighting, which is inserted into the uterus through the cervix to observe the uterine cavity, and through which instruments are introduced to perform surgical procedures. With a video camera attached, the surgeon views the operation on a TV monitor.

immune system A complex system of cellular and molecular components that comprise the body's defense system against foreign organisms and substances. It recognizes tissues that are "self" as distinguished from those that are "foreign." It utilizes antibodies and "killer cells" to attack foreign substances that it does not recognize as self.

incontinence Inability to control urination.

inflammation A swelling with redness, heat, and pain in any area as a result of irritation, trauma, infection, or abnormal immune function.

IUD (intrauterine device) An object inserted into the uterus, usually used for contraception. It can also be used to deliver hormones and medications directly into the uterus.

laparoscope A hollow tube with a fiberoptic lighting system, which can be inserted into the abdomen through a small incision to view internal organs.

Operating instruments can be inserted to perform surgery. A video camera can be attached for viewing the operation on a monitor screen.

laser vaporization A method of removing abnormal tissue by using a laser beam to vaporize it.

LEEP (loop electrosurgical excision procedure) A method of removing abnormal tissue from the cervix using a wire loop through which high frequency radio waves are transmitted.

LH (luteinizing hormone) A hormone produced by the pituitary gland that triggers ovulation and development of the corpus luteum from which progesterone is produced.

libido Level of sexual desire or sexual energy. Sex drive.

luteal phase The second half of the menstrual cycle from ovulation until the menstrual period begins. It is dominated by progesterone production in the corpus luteum after ovulation has taken place.

male hormones A group of hormones that produce masculine effects such as facial hair, body hair, acne, muscular development, deepening of the voice, and increased sexual desire.

malignant Cancerous.

mammogram X ray of the breast to screen for cancer.

menarche The initial onset of menstrual periods.

menopause The point in time when the final menstrual period has occurred.

metabolism The biotransformation of nutrients into tissue and useful energy by chemical processes utilizing oxygen, enzymes, vitamins, and other substances. *Anabolic metabolism* builds tissue, and *catabolic metabolism* expends energy.

myoma A benign muscle tumor in the uterus. Also known as a *fibroid*.

myomectomy Surgical removal of a myoma.

neural tube defects Abnormalities of the spinal column and head that occur as the embryo is forming. Abnormalities include *anencephaly* (absence of the brain), *spina bifida* (failure of the tail end of the spinal column to close), *meningomyelocele* (protrusion of membranes and spinal cord through a defect in the vertebrae), and *meningocele* (protrusion of membranes through a defect in the vertebrae or the skull).

neurotransmitters A variety of chemicals that facilitate the transmission of nerve impulses from nerve to nerve and between the brain and the rest of the body.

oncogene A gene capable with certain stimuli of converting normal cells into cancer cells. Normal genes may be converted to oncogenes under the influence of aging and external toxic dietary or environmental influences.

oophorectomy (ovariectomy) Surgical removal of one or both ovaries.

osteoporosis Loss of bone mass and strength from loss of bone minerals. Bones become porous and fracture easily.

ovarian failure The inability of the ovaries to respond to any hormonal stimulation. Menopause is the most common example.

ovarian stroma The supporting tissue or matrix of the ovary where androgens are produced.

ovaries The two female sex glands, also called *gonads*, situated on either side of the uterus, which contain eggs (ova) and produce the female sex hormones estrogen and progesterone. They also produce small amounts of the male hormone, testosterone.

ovulation Release of an egg from an ovarian follicle at mid-cycle.

parasympathetic nervous system The part of the autonomic nervous system that regulates body relaxation, growth, and repair. It regulates the heart, glands of the head and neck, intestines, and other structures with involuntary muscles. Its primary neurotransmitter is acetylcholine.

pelvic inflammatory disease (PID) Inflammation of pelvic organs, particularly the uterus and fallopian tubes, caused by infectious microorganisms. It typically occurs from sexually transmitted bacteria, fungi, and viruses.

perimenopause Describes the years from the time that hormone decline begins until the reproductive era is concluded at menopause. Hormonal decline begins in the mid- to late 30s, and menopause is typically at age 51.

pessary An oval shaped object inserted into the vagina to support a prolapsed uterus. It can also be a ring shaped object to deliver hormones to vaginal tissues.

pituitary gland A mushroom-shaped gland attached to the base of the brain by a stalk. It manufactures hormones (FSH, LH, TSH, ACTH, and others) that control the function of other hormone producing glands such as the ovaries, thyroid, and adrenals.

polycystic ovarian syndrome (PCO) A syndrome caused by an imbalance in the amount of LH and FSH released during the ovulatory cycle, resulting in development of multiple cysts in the ovaries due to arrested follicle growth.

postmenopause The entire time of life following the final menstrual period.

premature menopause The decline of ovarian hormones and permanent cessation of menstrual periods before the age of 40.

premenopause The years prior to menopause. See *perimenopause.*

premenstrual syndrome (PMS) A variable collection of physical and psychological/emotional symptoms recurring on a regular basis in the week or two preceding a menstrual period. Symptoms include mood disturbances, headache, bloating, weight gain.

progesterone The female hormone produced by the ovaries after ovulation that prepares the endometrium for reception of a fertilized egg and sustains pregnancy.

progestin A synthetic substance that has a similar effect on the body as natural progesterone produced by the ovaries. Progestin is used in HRT to protect the endometrium and in birth control pills to control bleeding.

prolactin A pituitary hormone that regulates lactation and milk production. High levels of prolactin inhibit ovulation.

prolapse The falling down or downward displacement of an organ such as the uterus.

proliferative endometrium The effect of estrogen on the lining of the uterus (endometrium) in its growth (proliferative) phase during the first half of the menstrual cycle.

proliferative phase The first half of the menstrual cycle during which estrogen causes proliferation (growth) of the endometrium.

prostaglandins Chemicals manufactured throughout the body that exert a hormonelike effect and influence involuntary muscular contraction (including the uterus), circulation, and inflammation.

regimen A strictly regulated scheme of medication, diet, or exercise designed to achieve certain ends.

salpingectomy Surgical removal of the fallopian tube.

secretory endometrium The lining of the uterus under the influence of progesterone during the second half of the menstrual cycle (the luteal phase). The secretory glands of the endometrium become filled with droplets of sugar, called glycogen, and the endometrium develops a rich blood supply in preparation for receiving a fertilized egg.

serotonin (5-HT) A potent derivative of the amino acid tryptophan, produced in the brain, nerve cells, intestine, and pineal gland. It functions in regulating mood, sleep, appetite, sexual desire, pain, repetitive thoughts, and repetitive actions. Dietary sources of tryptophan are animal and dairy products, whole grains, and beans.

sex hormones Female and male hormones produced from cholesterol molecules by the ovaries, adrenal glands, fat cells, and testicles. They include estrogen, progesterone, testosterone, and other weak androgens.

sympathetic nervous system The part of the autonomic nervous system that prepares the body to confront stressful situations through the release of stress hormones. Its primary neurotransmitters are norepinephrine and epinephrine.

syndrome A group of symptoms and physical signs that collectively characterize a disease.

testosterone The strongest male sex hormone produced in the testes, but also in small amounts by the ovarian stroma (interior supportive tissue of the ovary).

thyroid gland The endocrine gland at the base of the neck situated astride the trachea (wind pipe). Its hormones, thyroxine (T4) and triodothyronine (T3), regulate metabolism in all body tissues.

transdermal Through the skin. Transdermal skin patches are used to administer estrogen in HRT.

triglycerides (TG) A blood fat composed of three molecules of glycerol and derived mostly from diet, especially carbohydrates. TG is stored in fat cells and serves as a reservoir for making cholesterol. High TG levels combined with low HDL cholesterol are a significant risk factor for CVD in women.

TSH (thyroid stimulating hormone) The hormone produced by the pituitary gland that regulates the production and release of the thyroid hormones. TSH is high in *hypo*thyroidism and low in *hyper*thyroidism.

tubal ligation A surgical procedure to interrupt, obstruct, or tie off the fallopian tubes for permanent contraception.

tumor An abnormal growth, which may be benign or malignant.

ultrasound scan A scanning method to visualize internal organs and tissues using high frequency sound waves. It does not involve radiation.

urethra The canal that carries urine from the bladder to outside the body.

uterus The pelvic organ that carries and sustains a growing fetus during pregnancy.

vagina The genital passage from the uterus to the vulva. It is sufficiently muscular and elastic to accommodate the penis during sex or delivery of a baby.

vaginismus Spasm of the muscles around the opening of the vagina, making penetration during sexual intercourse either impossible or very painful. It can be caused by physical or psychological conditions.

vulva The female external genitalia.

REFERENCES CITED ✍

Chapter 1 BACKGROUND TALK

Sheehy, Gail. *The Silent Passage* (New York: Random House, 1991), p. 24.

Chapter 2 PERIMENOPAUSE: HOW IT HAPPENS

Speroff, Leon, R. H. Glass, and N. G. Kase. *Clinical Gynecologic Endocrinology and Infertility*, 4th ed. (Baltimore: Williams & Wilkins, 1989), p. 124.

Chapter 3 PERIMENOPAUSE: AS IT HAPPENS

Brown, J. Episiotomy and pelvic floor exercise for incontinence. *Audio Digest Obstetrics and Gynecology* 43 (November 21, 1996).

Campbell, S., and M. Whitehead. Estrogen therapy and the menopausal syndrome. *Clinical Obstetrics and Gynecology* 4 (1977): 31.

Chopra, Deepak. *Quantum Healing: Exploring the Frontier of Mind/Body Medicine.* New York: Bantam Books, 1993.

Gray, John. *Men Are from Mars, Women Are from Venus* (New York: HarperCollins, 1992), p. 15.

Kronenberg, Fredi. Hot flashes: epidemiology and physiology. *American Journal of the Academy of Science* (1990): 56–58.

———. "Menopausal Hot Flashes" (paper presented at the annual meeting of the North American Menopause Society, May 21, 1993).

Sheehy, Gail. *The Silent Passage* (New York: Random House, 1991), p. 113.

Wallace, J. P., et al. Changes in menstrual function, climacteric syndrome and serum concentrations of sex hormone in pre- and postmenopausal women following a moderate intensity training program. *Modern Science in Sports & Exercise* 14 (1982): 154.

Chapter 4 PERIMENOPAUSAL PREGNANCY

American College of Obstetricians & Gynecologists. "Estrogen replacement therapy in women with previously treated breast cancer" (A.C.O.G. Committee Opinion, no. 135, Washington, D.C., April 1994).

Darney, P. D. Oral contraceptives and upcoming slow-realease hormones. *Audio Digest Obstetrics and Gynecology* 43 (August 20, 1996).

Edge, V. L., and R. K. Laros. Pregnancy outcomes in nulliparous women aged 35 or older. *American Journal of Obstetrics & Gynecology* 168 (1993): 1881–85.

Chapter 5 CARDIOVASCULAR DISEASE

Bush, Trudy, et al. Lipid Research Clinics Follow-up Study. *Circulation* 75 (1987): 1102.

Clarkson, T. B., et al. *Cardiovascular Health and Disease in Women.* New York: W.B. Saunders, 1993.

Henderson, B. E., et al. Estrogen and cardiovascular disease. *American Journal of Obstetrics & Gynecology* 154 (1986): 1181.

Ravnikar, V., et al. Blood lipid levels in postmenopausal women on HRT. In *35th Annual Meeting, Society of Gynecologic Investigation* abstract no. 422 (1989).

Rexrode, K. M., and J. E. Manson. Antioxidants in cardiovascular disease prevention: Fact or fiction. *Menopausal Medicine* 6, no. 3 (1996): 8–12.

Speroff, Leon. Estrogen and cardiovascular disease. *Ob/Gyn Clinical Alert* 10 (1994): 86–88.

Stampfer, M. J., et al. The Nurses Health Study. *New England Journal of Medicine* 313 (1985): 1044.

Chapter 6 OSTEOPOROSIS

Abdella, H. I., et al. Prevention of bone mineral loss in postmenopausal women by norethisterone. *Obstetrics and Gynecology* 66 (1985): 789.

Avioli, L. V. Calcium and osteoporosis. *Annals of Review of Nutrition* 4 (1984): 471.

Cauley, J. A., et al. Prevention of osteoporotic fractures requires long term estrogen therapy. *Annals of Internal Medicine* 122 (1995): 9–16.

Christianson, C., et al. Uncoupling of bone formation and resorption by combined estrogen-progesterone therapy in postmenopausal osteoporosis. *Lancet* (1985): 800.

Felch, J. A., et al. Epidemiology of hip fractures in Norway. *Acta Orthopedica Scandinavia* 56 (1985): 12.

Hopper, J. L., and E. Seeman. Smoking and bone density. *New England Journal of Medicine* 330 (1994): 387–92.

Johnston, C. C., et al. Early menopausal changes in bone mass and sex steroids. *Journal of Clinical Endocrinology and Metabolism* 61 (1985): 905.

Kiel, D. P., et al. Hip fracture and the use of estrogens in postmenopausal women. The Framingham Study. *New England Journal of Medicine* 317 (1987): 1169.

Lindsay, R., et al. Bone response to termination of estrogen treatment. *Lancet* (1978): 1325.

Nachtigall, Lila, and Joan Heilman. *Estrogen: The Facts Can Change Your Life.* New York: Harper Perennial, 1995.

Prince, R., et al. Prevention of osteoporosis: A comparative study of exercise, calcium supplementation, and hormone replacement. *New England Journal of Science* 325 (1991): 1189–95.

Raisz, L. G. Bone formation and resorption in menopausal women using estrogen and androgen. *Journal of Endocrinology and Metabolism* 81 (1996): 37–73.

Riggs, B. L., et al. Effect of calcium regimen on vertebral fracture in postmenopausal osteoporosis. *New England Journal of Medicine* 306 (1982): 446.

Selby, P. L., et al. Early effects of ethinyl oestradiol and norethisterone treatment in postmenopausal women on bone resorption and calcium regulating hormones. *Clinical Science* 69 (1985) 265.

Speroff, Leon. Measuring bone density to screen for osteoporosis. *Ob/Gyn Clinical Alert* 2 (1995): 70–72.

———. Pamidronate protects bone. *Ob/Gyn Clinical Alert* 13, no. 10 (1997) 76–77.

Speroff, Leon, R. H. Glass, and N. G. Kase. *Clinical Gynecologic Endocrinology and Infertility*, 4th ed. (Baltimore: Williams & Wilkins, 1989), p. 138.

Theistz, G. Bone mass accumulation in adolescent and young adult women. *Journal of Clinical Endocrinology and Metabolism* 75 (1992): 1060–65.

Chapter 7 CANCER AND HORMONES

Ambrosone, C. B., et al. Cigarette smoking, N-acetyltransferase 2 genetic polymorphisms, and breast cancer risk. *Journal of the American Medical Association* 276 (1996): 1494–1501.

American College of Obstetricians and Gynecologists. Health Maintenance for Perimenopausal Women. *A.C.O.G. Technical Bulletin* no. 210 (August 1990).

Andrews, W. D. "Transition Years and Beyond" (paper presented at the 42nd annual meeting of the American College of Obstetricians and Gynecologists, 1994).

Gambrell, R. D., et al. Decreased incidence of breast cancer in postmenopausal estrogen-progesterone users. *Obstetrics and Gynecology* 62 (1983): 435.

———. Role of estrogen and progesterone in the etiology and prevention of endometrial cancer: a review. *American Journal of Obstetricians & Gynecologists* 146 (1983): 696.

Hankinson, S. E., G. A. Colditz, and D. J. Hunter. A quantitative assessment of oral contraceptive use and risk of ovarian cancer. *Obstetrics and Gynecology* 80 (1992): 708–14.

Henrich, J. B. The postmenopausal estrogen/breast cancer controversy. *Journal of the American Medical Association* 268 (1992): 1900–2.

Kaufman, D. W., et al. Noncontraceptive estrogen use and the risk of breast cancer. *Journal of the American Medical Association* 252 (1984): 63.

Melbye, M., et al. Induced abortion and the risk of breast cancer. *New England Journal of Medicine* 336 (1997): 81–85.

Michels, K. B. Birth weight as a risk for breast cancer. *Lancet* 348 (1996): 1542–46.

Newcomb, P. A., et al. *American Journal of Epidemiology* 142 (1995): 788–95.

Shattuck-Eidens, D., et al. A collaborative survey of 80 mutations of the BRCA-1 breast and ovarian cancer susceptibility gene. Implications for presymptomatic testing and screening. *Journal of the American Medical Association* 273 (1995): 535–41.

Speroff, Leon, R. H. Glass, and N. G. Kase. *Clinical Gynecologic Endocrinology and Infertility*, 4th ed. (New York: Williams & Wilkins, 1989), p. 148.

Tarone, Robert. Breast cancer death rate continues to decline. *News from the National Cancer Institute* (July 1996).

W.H.O. collaborative study of neoplasia and steroid contraceptives. Breast cancer, cervical cancer and medroxyprogesterone acetate. *Lancet* (1984): 1207.

Wingo, P. A., et al. The risk of breast cancer in postmenopausal women who have used estrogen replacement therapy. *Journal of the American Medical Association* 257 (1987): 209.

Chapter 8 VISIBLE CHANGES

Cauley, J. A., et al. The decline of grip strength in menopause: relationship to physical activity, estrogen use, and anthropometric factors. *Journal of Chronic Disease* 40 (1987): 115.

Fantl, J. A., et al. *Obstetrics & Gynecology* 88 (1996): 745–49.

Fulton, J. E., G. Pluwig, and A. M. Kilgman. The effect of chocolate on acne vulgaris. *Journal of the American Medical Association* 210 (1996): 2071–74.

Mishell, D. R. Menopause: Timing and symptoms. *Contemporary Ob/Gyn* (November 1995): 11–17.

Chapter 9 SEX AFTER MENOPAUSE

Bachman, Gloria. "Sexual Problems during Menopause" (paper presented at the Menopausal Syndrome Symposium, Scottsdale, Ariz., January 27, 1990).

Edelman, Deborah. *Sex in the Golden Years*. New York: Donald I. Fine, 1992.

Koster, A. Changed life anticipations, attitudes and experiences among middle-aged Danish women. *Health Care for Women International* 12 (1991): 1.

Masters, Virginia, and William Johnson. *Human Sexual Inadequacy*. Boston: Little, Brown, 1970.

Nachtigall, Lila, and Joan Heilman. *Estrogen: The Facts Can Save Your Life* (New York: Harper/Perennial, 1995), p. 112.

Ploutte, L., and P. Conen. *Comprehensive Management of Menopause* (London: Springer-Verlag, 1994), p. 297–308.

Chapter 11 HORMONE REPLACEMENT THERAPY (HRT)

American College of Obstetricians & Gynecologists. Hormone Replacement Therapy. *A.C.O.G. Technical Bulletin* no. 166 (1992).

Araneo, B. A., et al. DHEAS as an effective adjuvant in elderly humans: Proof-of-principle studies. *Annals of the New York Academy of Science* 774 (1995): 332–48.

Bates, G. W., et al. Dehydroepiandrosterone attenuates study-induced declines in insulin sensitivity in postmenopausal women. *Annals of the New York Academy of Science* 774 (1995): 291–93.

Baulieu, E. Dehydroepiandrosterone (DHEA) is a neuroactive neurosteroid. *Annals of the New York Academy of Science* 774 (1995): 82–110.

Brody, J. "Drug Researchers Working to Design Customized Estrogen." *New York Times*, March 4, 1997.

Ettinger, B., et al. Postmenopausal bone loss is prevented by treatment with low-dose estrogen with calcium. *Annals of Internal Medicine* 106 (1987): 40.

Felson, D. T., et al. Hormone replacement therapy compliance. *New England Journal of Medicine* 329 (1993): 1141–46.

Grady, D., et al. Hormone replacement therapy and endometrial cancer risk: a meta-analysis. *Obstetrics & Gynecology* 85 (1995): 304.

Hargrove, J. T., et al. Menopausal hormone replacement therapy with continuous daily micronized estradiol and progesterone. *Obstetrics & Gynecology* 23 (1989): 606.

Lindheim, S. R., et al. Estrogen and stress. *Journal Obstet. Invest.* 1 (1994): 79–83.

Michels, K. B., et al. Birth weight as a factor for breast cancer. *Lancet* 348 (1996): 1542–46.

Ornish, Dean. *Reversing Heart Disease.* New York: Ballantine Books, 1990.

Paganinni-Hill, A., and V. W. Henderson. Estrogen and Alzheimer's disease. *American Journal of Epidemiology* 140 (1994): 256–61.

Parsons, Anna. Sonography: a new method to evaluate the endometrium. *Menopausal Medicine* 1 (1993): 9–11.

Robinson, D., et al. Estrogen and memory. *Journal of the American Geriatric Society* 42 (1994): 919–22.

Schwartz, A. Dehydroepiandrosterone (DHEA) and aging. *Annals of the New York Academy of Science* 774 (1995): 121–27.

Speroff, Leon. Estrogen and cardiovascular disease. *Ob/Gyn Clinical Alert* 10 (1994): 86–88.

———. Postmenopausal hormone therapy and endometrial cancer. *Ob/Gyn Clinical Alert* 12 (1997): 95–96.

Wolkowitz, O. M., et al. Antidepressant and cognition-enhancing effects of DHEA in major depression. *Annals of the New York Academy of Science* 774 (1995): 337–39.

Writing Group for the PEPI Trial. *Journal of the American Medical Association* 273 (1995): 199–208.

Chapter 12 ALTERNATIVE THERAPIES

Aldercreutz, H., et al. Dietary phyto-estrogens and the menopause in Japan. *Lancet* 339 (1992): 1233.

Bienfield, H., and E. Korngold. *Between Heaven and Earth: A Guide to Chinese Medicine.* New York: Ballantine Books, 1991.

Bouchayer, R. Alternative medicines: a general approach to the French situation. *Comprehensive Medical Research* 4 (1990): 4–8.

Chopra, Deepak. *Quantum Healing: Exploring the Frontier of Mind/Body Medicine.* New York: Bantam Books, 1990.

Khoo, S. K., C. Munro, and D. Battistta. Evening primrose oil and treatment of PMS. *Medical Journal of Australia* 153 (1990): 189–92.

Kleijmen, J. Evening primrose oil currently used in many conditions with little justification. *British Medical Journal* 309 (1994): 824–25.

Tyler, V. E. The bright side of black cohosh. *Prevention* 4 (1997): 76–79.

Ullman, D. *Discovering Homeopathic Medicine for the 21st Century*. Berkeley: North Atlantic Books, 1991.

Chapter 13   STRESS MANAGEMENT

American College of Obstetricians & Gynecologists. Stress in the Practice of Obstetrics and Gynecology. *A.C.O.G. Technical Bulletin* no. 149 (1990).

Benson, H., and W. Proctor. *Beyond the Relaxation Response*. New York: Time Books, 1984.

Benson, H., and E. Stuart. *The Wellness Book*. New York: Simon & Schuster, 1992.

Choruso, G. P., and P. W. Gold. The concept of stress and stress systems disorders: overview of physical and behavioral homeostasis. *Journal of the American Medical Association* 267 (1992): 1244–52.

Giordano D. A., G. S. Everly, and D. E. Dusek. *Controlling Stress and Tension System Disorders: A Holistic Approach*, 4th ed. New York: Prentice Hall, 1993.

Kaufman, S. "How Creativity Can Take Wing at the Edge of Chaos." Interview by Thomas Petzinger, Jr. *Wall Street Journal*, October 18, 1996, B-1.

Kobasa, S., S. Maddi, and S. Kahn. Hardiness and Health: A Prospective Study. *Journal of Personality and Social Psychology* 42 (1982): 168–77.

Landau, Carol, M. G. Cyr, and A. W. Moulton. *The Complete Book of Menopause* (New York: G.P. Putnam, 1994), p. 221.

Moyers, Bill. *Healing and the Mind*. New York: Bantam, Doubleday Dell, 1993.

Wilde, L. "Humor: Rx for Healing, Health, and Happiness" (presentation at Rogue Valley Medical Center, Medford, Oreg., April 22, 1997).

Yerkes, R. M., and J. D. Dodson. The relation of strength of stimulus to rapidity of habit-formation. *Journal of Comparative Neurology and Psychology* 18 (1989): 459–82.

Chapter 14   FITNESS

Abenhaim, J., et al. Appetite suppressant drugs and the risk of pulmonary hypertension. *New England Journal of Medicine* 335 (1996): 609–15.

American College of Obstetricians & Gynecologists. Women and Exercise. *A.C.O.G. Technical Bulletin* no. 149 (1990).

Blair, S. N., et al. Physical fitness and all-cause mortality: a prospective study of healthy men and women. *Journal of the American Medical Association* 262 (1989): 2395–401.

Cone, Faye Kitchener. *Making Sense of Menopause* (New York: Simon & Schuster, 1993), p. 199.

Connor, S., and W. Connor. *The New American Diet System*. New York: Simon & Schuster, 1991.

Franklin, B. A. Aerobic exercise training programs for the upper body. *Medical Science in Sports and Exercise* 21 (1989): S141–48.

Institute of Medicine. *Improving America's Diet and Health: From Recommendation to Action*. National Academy Press, 1991.

Kowalski, R. E. *The Eight-Week Cholesterol Cure: How to Lower Your Blood Cholesterol by Up to 40% Without Drugs or Deprivation*, rev. ed. (New York: Harper & Row, 1990), p. 282.

Ojeda, L. *Menopause Without Medicine*. Alameda, Calif.: Hunter House, 1995.

Ornish, Dean. *Reversing Heart Disease*. New York: Ballantine Books, 1990.

Rikki, R. "Health Guide 1995." Interview by S. Brink. *U.S. News and World Report*, May 15, 1995, 75–84.

von Schacky, C. Prophylaxis of atherosclerosis with marine omega-3 fatty acids. *Annals of Internal Medicine* 107 (1987): 890–99.

Chapter 15 MENOPAUSE FROM OTHER CAUSES

Carlson, K. J. Indications for hysterectomy. *New England Journal of Medicine* 328 (1993): 856–60.

Cutler, Winnifred, and Ramon Celso-Garcia. *Menopause: A Guide for Women and the Men Who Love Them* (New York: W. W. Norton, 1992), p. 216.

Feeney, D. D., et al. Fate of the ovaries after hysterectomy and ovarian transposition. *Gynecologic Oncology* 56 (1995): 3–7.

Loft, N. L. Ovarian function after premenopausal hysterectomy. *Ugeskrift for Laeger* 155 (1993): 3818–22.

Ravina, J. H., et al. Arterial embolisation to treat uterine myomata. *Lancet* 346 (1995): 671–72.

Ravnikar, V. Physiology and treatment of hot flashes. *Obstetrics & Gynecology* 75 (1990): 38–85.

Rector, R. C. Chronic pelvic pain. *Clinical Ob/Gyn* 33 (1990): 117.

Sherwin, B., and M. Gelfand. Sex steroids and effect in the surgical menopause: a double blind, cross-over study. *Psychoneuroendocrinology* 3 (1985): 325–35.

Utian, W., and R. Jacobwitz. *Managing Your Menopause*. New York: Prentice Hall, 1990.

Chapter 17 JUST FOR MEN: ANDROPAUSE AND MENOPAUSE

Barbach, Lonnie. *The Pause: Positive Approaches to Menopause* (New York: Signet Books, 1993), p. 239.

Utian, Wulf, and Ruth Jacobwitz. *Managing Your Menopause* (New York: Prentice Hall, 1990), p. 157.

Chapter 18 THE NEXT THIRD

Sheehy, Gail. *New Passages*. New York, Random House, 1995.

INDEX

The letter *f* following a page reference indicates an illustration. The letter *t* following a page reference indicates a table.